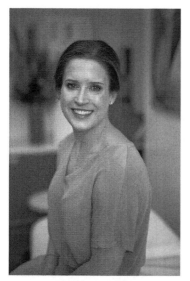

Photo by Maryanne Scott

Dr Natalia Spierings, BSc MBBS MRCP(UK) MRCP(Derm) MBA MSc, is a UK-trained Consultant Dermatologist, having done her medical, junior doctor and dermatology training at St George's, University of London. As well as having a master's degree in aesthetic medicine from Queen Mary, University of London, Dr Spierings has completed a fellowship in Mohs Micrographic and Dermatological Surgery at the Royal Victoria Infirmary in Newcastle and her subspeciality area of expertise is the diagnosis and management of skin cancer as well as skin surgery. You can see her in action on Channel 5's *Skin A&E*, now in its third season. When she is not seeing patients or providing evidence-based skincare advice on social media, you can find her lifting weights in the gym.

To my parents, Maria and Egilius Spierings

Skin*telligent*

What you really need to know to get great skin

Dr Natalia Spierings
CONSULTANT DERMATOLOGIST

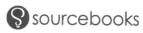 sourcebooks

Copyright © 2022 by Dr. Natalia Spierings
Illustrations copyright © 2022 by Charlotte Willcox
Cover design by Nic&Lou

Sourcebooks and the colophon are registered trademarks of Sourcebooks.

All rights reserved. No part of this book may be reproduced in any form or by
any electronic or mechanical means including information storage and retrieval
systems—except in the case of brief quotations embodied in critical articles or
reviews—without permission in writing from its publisher, Sourcebooks.

This publication is designed to provide accurate and authoritative information
in regard to the subject matter covered. It is sold with the understanding
that the publisher is not engaged in rendering legal, accounting, or other
professional service. If legal advice or other expert assistance is required,
the services of a competent professional person should be sought. —*From
a Declaration of Principles Jointly Adopted by a Committee of the American
Bar Association and a Committee of Publishers and Associations*

Published by Sourcebooks
P.O. Box 4410, Naperville, Illinois 60567-4410
(630) 961-3900
sourcebooks.com

Originally published in 2022 in Great Britain by Vermilion, an imprint of
Ebury Publishing, part of the Penguin Random House group of companies.

Cataloging-in-Publication Data is on file with the Library of Congress.

Printed and bound in the United States of America.
POD

Contents

Introduction   1

Part 1: How Skin Works   **11**

   1   The Structure of the Skin   13
   2   The Myth of the Skin 'Type'   33
   3   How Skin Changes as We Age   47

Part 2: How Skincare Works (Or Doesn't)   **59**

   4   Facial Cleansers and Moisturisers   63
   5   Sunscreen   87
   6   Skincare Products You Don't Need   97

Part 3: Unravelling Big Skincare Ingredient Claims **111**

   7   Vitamin A   121
   8   Hydroquinone   133
   9   Vitamin C   141
  10   Acids   147
  11   Other Common Cosmetic Ingredients   153

**Part 4: How to Treat the Most Common Facial
           Skin Diseases**   **159**

  12   Acne Vulgaris   163
  13   Rosacea   201
  14   Dermatitis   215
  15   Melasma and Facial Hyperpigmentation   221

Part 5: How to Tackle Common Aesthetic Concerns   **231**

  16   Fine Lines and Wrinkles   233
  17   Dark Under-Eye Circles   241

18 Unwanted or Excess Facial Hair   245
19 Skin 'Rejuvenation'   259

Final Words   273

Appendix: How to Choose a Dermatologist   277
Acknowledgements   279
References   281
Index   307

Introduction

This is not a book about what the 'best' or 'worst' skincare brands are. I am not going to tell you to double cleanse, use a toner, exfoliate and moisturise twice a day (oh, and don't forget the eye cream, of course!). There are no lists of brand and product recommendations at the end of each chapter or complicated, detailed 'skincare routines'.

What I *will* do is present you with the science and the evidence (and critically appraise it), as well as the history behind the concept of 'skincare' in its modern iteration, giving you all the information you need to get the right treatment for the most common facial skin problems – from pimples and pigmentation to wrinkles and oily skin.

The bottom line – and what I will emphasise throughout this book – is that **facial skin health and disease is very much a medical problem, not merely a cosmetic issue**. And 99 per cent of skincare products should be viewed as luxury goods, not necessities (as you will soon discover, there is no such thing as 'essential' skincare). After all, the skin is an organ and has many important functions aside from helping us look good (or sometimes bad, if skin disease isn't managed well). As a society we need to stop taking our skincare advice from people whose motives for recommending specific products are almost entirely financially driven; this includes skincare companies, journalists, bloggers, beauty therapists, YouTubers and even some medical professionals. I refer to this seemingly diverse group of people collectively as 'Big Skincare', but more on that later.

As a doctor, I took an oath and the most important part of

that oath is honesty and integrity; my reputation is based on trust and that trust derives from the fact that I always strive to tell the truth about everything from serums to skin cancer. My patients – and now you – know that I have their best interests at heart. Skin disease is devastating and frustrating for so many people, so it cannot and should not be trivialised by a ten-step skincare plan, a series of facials or a 'magic' cream. Above all else, when providing healthcare, there is no room for greed: maximising personal financial gain does not come before optimising patient outcomes. For me, it never has and it never will.

The bottom line: I didn't become a doctor as part of a 'get rich quick' scheme!

So, what *is* the truth behind skincare? Are expensive products better than cheap ones? Do you really need to cleanse, tone and moisturise twice a day to have 'great' skin? Do you need eye cream to prevent wrinkles around your eyes when you get older? Are facials important? Do you have to wear sunscreen all day, every day, even indoors? What's the best way to treat pimples? Are treatments for pigmentation safe? These are some of the questions I receive every day from my patients – and my goal is to give you the answers to all of these (and many more) in this book so you have the tools and knowledge to be able to make an informed decision about what skincare products you want to spend your time and money on, based on what you like to use, your specific skin situation, the science and your budget.

WHO AM I?

I am a UK-trained, half-Dutch (my dad), half-Polish (my mum), USA-bred (Boston) Consultant Dermatologist. Fortunately, my ability to practise clinical medicine far exceeds my language skills (I really only speak English properly, putting my heritage and my parents to shame).

I love learning and understanding the minutiae of science – how cells work, how the immune system works. To be more precise: I like the process and challenge of learning (I'm fairly happy to learn about anything, from cooking to politics to religion). I like gaining knowledge. But I don't like to learn things just for the sake of it. There must be a practical application, a reason. And that's why I chose to study medicine over any of the sciences.

SKINTELLIGENT FACT:

Doc, why do you sound like an American?

If I had £1 for every time a patient asked me this question . . .

I was born in Rotterdam, the Netherlands on a sparkling, sunny day in March 1981. I enjoyed a childhood of cycling and visiting the biggest zoo in Europe (in Blijdorp – literally 'Happy Village') until the age of six when my dad got offered a job in Boston, Massachusetts and we moved. It was only meant to be for 2 years, but we all know how these things go: almost 40 years later, and my parents still live in Boston. Hence I have an American accent. I have an older brother who is married with two kids and lives in Rotterdam (in the Happy Village). When I was 18, I moved back to Holland to finish up my high-school education in The Hague and was encouraged to apply to medical school in the UK. So I did. And I got into St George's in London and decided to move without ever having been to the UK before. I liked it, so I stayed – and ended up doing all my junior doctor training as well as my dermatology training at St George's.

My approach to health and skincare

I was a fat child and I spent my teenage years, my twenties and well into my thirties trying to be 'not fat'. I read every book, every fitness magazine; I tried every diet, every exercise programme; I read the blogs, the scientific papers; I tried the pills, the programmes, the shakes. Keto, Atkins, South Beach, paleo, vegan, intermittent fasting, bulletproof coffee – you name it, I tried it. Despite all this time, effort and money spent, I never got the body I wanted.

Then, after almost 35 years of this, I stumbled upon someone who told me that everything I had learnt and religiously followed about diet, exercise and weight loss was absolute nonsense: Menno Henselmans. Using an evidence-based approach, Menno made me see sense and question everything I had thought was true about weight loss. And you can predict what happened: I got there. I got the body I never thought I would have. But it took me letting go of all the marketing gimmicks I had believed for so many years and just focusing on what is simple, true, logical and based in science. Menno didn't get me to buy protein powder or eat fake food or use supplements; he simplified my life and just said it how it is. He told me to train properly with heavy weights and correct form and to not eat junk food; to sleep at least eight hours a night; to reduce my stress levels; to eat enough of the right foods to feel satiated . . . and to do it consistently.

Only recently have I realised the similarity between the way Menno views fat loss and the way I view skincare. His number-one goal is to get people muscular and lean. My number-one goal is to get people the best skin of their lives. And we approach our goals in exactly the same way: by cutting out the junk and helping our clients/patients understand the facts to give them the knowledge and therefore the confidence to go against the mainstream 'noise' that envelops and confuses these topics in order to reach their goals.

I know it sounds like a cliché, but I really love to help

people. And, as a doctor, I have committed my life to doing so in the most practical way possible. Even on the hardest days, I remind myself that I have been given a gift and I should not take that for granted or take advantage of the trust people have in me because of my professional title. My job is to help people feel better, not sell them useless lotions or potions or tell them things just to please them or avoid controversy. It is my job to provide ethical, honest, evidence-based care. My mission is to get people great skin by using my in-depth understanding of skin physiology and pathology and my vast clinical experience – and this book allows me to reach all those people who can't come and see me in my clinic.

SKINTELLIGENT FACT:

I practise evidence-based skincare

It might at first glance look like an oxymoron, but it's not – it's how I approach the confusing world of cosmetic skincare: by looking for good-quality evidence. And there isn't very much of it if we define 'evidence' as being randomised controlled clinical trials. To determine if it's 'good-quality', I then analyse the trial by looking at the methodology (how they did it) and the statistical analysis (how they made the numbers show what they show).

The number-one issue in dermatology and skincare over the past 20 or so years of research is that so many of the trials are industry-sponsored (by 'industry' I mean Big Skincare) and therefore probably untrustworthy. 'Industry-sponsored' is the equivalent of you baking a cake for a baking competition and also being the taste-tester and the judge. Who do you think is going to win the competition, especially if winning could make you millions of pounds in cash? Because of this, I have expanded the definition of 'evidence-based skincare' to include the basic science aspect of skin as well as clinical experience. Luckily, what we do have is a great deal of in-depth research into how skin actually works in health and disease. Some of the best basic science research into skin was done back in the 1980s and it is really eye-opening. Clinical experience is very valuable in areas of medicine where we don't have high-quality evidence or research – and skincare is a great example. But I am not talking about one anecdotal experience; I am talking about experience over time that is observed by an astute clinician who has a sound knowledge base in first principles and can think laterally. And that is what I aim to do every day, with every patient I see.

WHO AND WHAT IS 'BIG SKINCARE'?

I define 'Big Skincare' as follows:

BIG SKINCARE: noun
The individuals, groups, companies and corporations that are involved in the *for-profit* creation, marketing, promotion, sales and confusion relating to skincare and cosmetic skincare products. Estimated total value of Big Skincare as a whole by 2025: US$189.3 billion.[1]

The skincare industry is a colossal cultural force and its sheer size and influence create challenges for anyone seeking to get to the truth about the products it makes and promotes.

Contradictory statements are a dime a dozen in the skincare

arena: double cleanse or not cleanse at all? Is toner necessary or not? Are vitamin C serums a must or totally pointless? Do you need to take a collagen supplement? To find impartial information is virtually impossible – everyone seemingly has an ulterior motive and that ulterior motive is normally financially driven.

For the majority of skincare products, there is either no data or only small studies produced by the proponents of the product. Of course, this is understandable; major medicine and cosmetic regulating bodies in the world are quite clear about what a cosmetic is and what it isn't, so strong scientific evidence for efficacy is completely unnecessary, as long as the skincare industry stays on the correct side of marketing gibberish. People will still buy the extortionately priced, caviar-laced, gold-flecked moisturiser used by an A-list celebrity regardless of any proof of efficacy. Additionally, there are people whose entire careers are based on 'reviewing' and 'selling' skincare products via social media, and they make a fortune from affiliate links and 'paid promotions'. Some of these people are doctors, but most of them are journalists or beauticians. Regardless of background, they are all puppets of the skincare industry – salespeople disguised as 'experts'. And they make a living by selling you pseudoscience nonsense. Let's refer to them collectively as 'skincare influencers'.

The popular media and social media don't help either. It is rare to come across a magazine article or online video stating that nothing works – that doesn't lend itself to increasing followers, monetising your social media account or getting a spot on morning television.

Many patients come to see me because they are confused skincare consumers who have lost trust in Big Skincare; often this is simply because they have bought and used many expensive or heavily marketed products to tackle specific problems, like pigmentation, and yet their skin looks the same as it did before shelling out hundreds of pounds on a plethora of cleansers, serums, toners, eye creams, exfoliants and masks.

To find an expert who can provide a reasonably independent view of the alleged benefits of the myriad skincare products and services available is extremely challenging. But I will state now, at the outset, that **I have no financial motivation with regards to skincare**. I am absolutely not a 'skincare influencer' (perhaps quite the opposite – I'm more of a skincare 'dissenter'). I don't work with or do paid partnerships with any skincare company or brand. I don't have any 'affiliate links' floating around my social media. My online content is not sponsored by anyone. I try very hard to maintain my impartiality and to approach all skincare products and treatments with logic and common sense.

So my skincare recommendations are always based on basic skin science first and foremost, combined with my extensive clinical experience from seeing thousands of patients a year and what will actually help. That's why some of my explanations can be a little complicated, but there is no way around that because *skin is complicated*. Oversimplifying skin is one of the biggest problems with cosmetic skincare and has caused a lot of issues for the skincare-buying public, patients and doctors. With this book, I want to challenge you to take a step back from the noise of 'Big Skincare' so you can really understand your skin and how to best look after it – it's finally time for unbiased, accurate information from someone who is on your side. Let me help you become not only an informed skincare consumer but also truly intelligent about your skin. **It's time for you to become Skintelligent.**

HOW TO USE THIS BOOK

In Part 1, we will explore each layer of the skin in detail, as well as the various skin appendages (like oil glands and hair follicles), touching on fundamental facts and science-based details, focusing on the most up-to-date, evidence-based information available and relating it back as much as possible to you and your skin. We'll also cover the myth of skin 'types', how skin ages in general and how the signs of skin ageing develop.

In Part 2 we will take a deep dive into how skincare works, starting with the three 'basic' skincare steps of facial cleansing, moisturising and sunscreen use. If you are totally new to skincare, this will help you decide whether using these types of products is right for you, and what using them actually does for your skin. I will then take you through the skincare products you almost certainly don't need so you can save your money and your skin!

Part 3 is all about unravelling Big Skincare claims by looking at the main ingredients found in skincare, often referred to as 'actives'. The scientific evidence for each ingredient is critically appraised and paired with my clinical experience of their efficacy (or lack thereof!) so you can make an informed decision about what may be right for you and your skin.

Parts 4 and 5 give my evidence- and experience-based recommendations for the treatment of the most common facial skin diseases as well as aesthetic concerns – everything from acne to sebaceous filaments to dark under-eye circles and excess facial hair.

Though I like to read books from front to back in a logical order, this book is totally amenable to 'skipping around' to what interests you the most – whether that's melasma, acne vulgaris or the best moisturiser to use. However, try to at least dip into Part 1 before you get started as that is the foundation of the book and will help you get the most out of it.

SKINCARE TERMINOLOGY

When discussing skincare, terminology is important. When I talk about skincare, I am referring to 'cosmetic skincare' - the stuff you buy at a department store or in the aisles of a pharmacy or drug store (or online, of course). I also refer to these products as 'adjuvant' skincare - products you use *alongside* a specific treatment.

I refer to skincare used to treat skin disease or correct or prevent a problem as 'treatments'. Most treatments (but not all) are prescribed by a doctor and are almost always very specific to one skin ailment or problem. I refer to treatments that you apply to your skin (like creams or ointments) as 'topical' treatments. 'Systemic' treatments are pills you swallow. 'Injectable' treatments are those that are injected directly into the skin.

PART 1

How Skin Works

No one dies of old skin! The skin never really wears out or falls off . . . we are all packaged to the very end.

Dr Arthur Balin and Dr Albert Kligman in
Aging and the Skin[1]

A recent survey of British skincare purchasing habits found that the average woman spends £570 a year on skincare and 19 minutes on a skincare routine every single day.[2] That's over two hours a week. And the questions that plague so many of us when it comes to skincare are still left unanswered: Am I doing the right thing? Should I be using a different cleanser/moisturiser/serum? Is what I am using actually working? Why do I still have spots/pigmentation/wrinkles/dryness?

Clearly, the cosmetic skincare industry is booming and will continue to grow. At the same time, modern skincare consumers are demonstrating an increasing appetite for education and information relating to the products they are being sold. However, a brief, simplistic overview of the science of skin is patronising and generally unhelpful, and certainly does not make you a more informed patient or consumer. Let's do this differently.

Let's go back to biology – and immunology and physiology and chemistry – class so you can gain some real knowledge and understanding, and get answers to and, more importantly, thorough explanations for all your many skincare questions.

The first step is to understand how your skin actually works – beyond oversimplified basics. What is the skin barrier? How does it work? What really makes up the dermis? In this section, I am therefore going to focus on the parts of the skin that are relevant to understanding skincare. Only when you understand these things can you delve into how skincare works (or doesn't). Then, armed with that knowledge, you can take the correct steps to managing any skin issues you may have with a cost-effective, efficient, common-sense approach. Let's take away the confusion and the pseudoscience gibberish and make you Skintelligent.

1

The Structure of the Skin

We are going to begin our journey through the structure and function of the skin from the top – the stratum corneum – and get right down to the fat (the subcutaneous tissue, that is). I think it is incredibly important to get a handle on the fundamentals of skin because these terms and ideas are used so often by Big Skincare to market and sell products. If you understand them, you will be able to appreciate how so much of what is sold to you doesn't really make much sense.

First up though, we need to discuss what normal skin is. As you can probably see by looking around you, there is a range of what people consider to be 'normal skin' throughout the world. However, for the purpose of this book, it does need a definition. When I am dealing with a patient, here is how I define 'normal skin': it has a 'regularly irregular' surface – take a second to reread that. Regularly irregular. The surface of the skin is composed of skin cells, with intervening hairs, sweat ducts and oil glands. It is gently undulating, but still reflects light in a way that makes it appear relatively smooth. Normal skin can be mildly pigmented (with brown spots on it like freckles) and it can range in colour from very pale, almost translucent white, to very dark brown. It can also be slightly red- or yellow-tinged, depending on your ethnic background or any skin issues that may be present.

Normal skin is slightly oily in the centre of the face and perhaps a little drier towards the outside. This is what people refer to as 'combination' skin – when in fact we all have combination skin to a certain degree. Some people are just oilier in their mid-face area (the 'T zone').

As time passes and we chronologically age and are exposed to the world around us (sun, smoking, stress), skin changes, though to me it still stays within a range of 'normal' (as long as no skin disease is present) with fine lines and deeper lines developing around the eyes, the mouth and the forehead. Pigmentation spots can appear and get darker and little blood vessels can become more prominent on the nose and cheeks of lighter-skinned people. These are all still normal changes – though we may not like them!

Many patients come to see me worrying that their skin barrier is 'weak' or 'damaged' and looking for advice on how to 'repair' it, when in fact they have perfectly normal, healthy skin. The fact is that if you have normal, healthy skin, your skin barrier is certainly intact and using too many products intended to 'strengthen' it can do more harm than good. Let's understand why, by exploring the stratum corneum's structure and function.

THE STRATUM CORNEUM

To understand how skincare products do or do not 'work' (and to make sense of the marketing jargon surrounding each and every lotion, potion and ingredient), we need to make sense of the stratum corneum. The stratum corneum is the very top of the skin – it's the part you see and feel.

The thickness of the stratum corneum ranges from 10 to 20μm – that's the thickness of clingfilm – and it contains 15 per cent water. At a very basic level, the stratum corneum is the one structure in our bodies that allows us to live on the dry earth because it seals water into our bodies – and our bodies are 60 per cent water! Traditionally, it has been viewed as a two-way seal, hence it is often referred to as the skin 'barrier'. And Big Skincare goes on about the skin barrier incessantly!

But this is a vast oversimplification. The stratum corneum is so much more than just a brick wall: it is an active structure that attracts and holds on to moisture for hydration, maintains its health and controls its shedding cycle. In other words, it is more like a medieval fortress, full of life and activity, that can fully support itself, rather than a lifeless barrier. Each cell of the stratum corneum has a purpose and a function.

That being said, **probably the most important function of the stratum corneum is to keep water inside the skin.** 'Transepidermal water loss' (TEWL) is the amount of water that evaporates through the skin to the external environment. The average TEWL through your skin is about 300–400ml per day, but this can be affected by environmental and internal factors. For example, in high-humidity climates, the amount of water loss will decrease.[1]

> *Transepidermal water loss (TEWL)*: the amount of water that passively evaporates through the skin to the external environment.

The stratum corneum is made up of long, flattened cells called 'corneocytes'. The stratum corneum is 14–16 corneocytes thick.[2] Each corneocyte is densely packed with keratin protein and has a well-defined sturdy envelope surrounding it. The corneocytes are tightly bound together, separated only by narrow spaces.

> *Corneocyte*: a flattened dead cell that has lost its nucleus and sits at the top of the skin, in the stratum corneum layer.

The corneocytes are held together by structures called 'corneodesmosomes' – think of it like Blu-Tack. These little rivets between the cells need to be digested away by enzymes to allow the very top of the stratum corneum to shed. Cells are constantly being shed from the top of your skin and replaced by others from underneath – a process known as 'desquamation'. This is happening without you being aware of it; healthy skin sheds its top layer without any noticeable skin flakiness or peeling and without the need for 'regular exfoliation' – another myth Big Skincare has propagated that has no basis in how skin actually works.[3]

The bottom line: You can ditch the grainy scrubs – your stratum corneum will be much happier!

The corneocyte envelopes are made up of a group of different proteins that interact to provide stability and strength. These proteins, such as fillagrin and involucrin, are also known as 'natural moisturising factors' (NMFs) – another name and concept that Big Skincare has grabbed on to; you can now buy skincare products made of NMFs, but applying these proteins to your skin doesn't mean they somehow make their way into the corneocyte envelope and strengthen it – that's just not possible because each corneoctye envelope is wrapped in its own lipid (fat) envelope that helps the corneocytes stay tightly packed together, but also provides a barrier to the passage of water into and out of the corneocyte.[4]

Many factors can influence the NMFs in the corneocytes.[5] Routine cleansing, for example, can wash out soluble NMFs in the stratum corneum. Low humidity in the environment, as well as sun exposure, can impair the function of the enzymes that break down filaggrin into its NMF components, therefore leading to a dry skin surface. There is also an age-related decline in the amount of NMFs in the skin. People who don't produce enough NMFs or don't produce them at all have serious skin diseases – like ichthyosis vulgaris or atopic dermatitis – but these people don't benefit from applying NMFs to their skin either (obviously).

The bottom line: You do not need to purchase a serum made of NMFs!

One of the critical functions of water in the stratum corneum is that it participates in the processes required for the corneo-cytes to desquamate, or shed, from the top of the skin. If the water content of the stratum corneum goes below a critical level, the enzymes that allow the skin cells to shed normally are impaired, leading to the corneocytes sticking together and clumping on the skin surface. We see and feel this as skin roughness, dryness, scaling and flaking. The stratum corneum water content can also be lowered due to a variety of reasons, including low humidity, sun exposure and the use of skin cleansers containing surfactants ('surface-active' substances).[6]

The narrow spaces between the corneocytes are long, winding pathways and that is how substances pass in and out of the skin. This space is made up of fats referred to as a 'lipid matrix' (see below).[7]

In summary, the stratum corneum is made up of water- and protein-filled flattened cells sitting in a bed of fat. Below is an illustration of what this looks like – however, this is only a graphic and does not do justice to how extraordinarily complex the stratum corneum is!

Across the 14–16 cells of the stratum corneum exists a pH gradient. At the bottom of the stratum corneum, the pH is about 7 (neutral) and it goes to an acidic 5 at the top. This acidic skin surface is called the 'acid mantle', which is a term used and abused by Big Skincare to sell products like cleansers that are meant to simultaneously protect and restore the pH of the skin surface.[8] Originally, the reason we have an acid skin surface was thought to be purely as a defence mechanism against invading organisms like bacteria. But, through the years, science has shown that pH has a profound effect on the way a healthy stratum corneum is created and maintained. Key enzymes function only at specific pH levels in the skin, so it is important to think of skin pH as a signalling system as well as a defence mechanism. When skin becomes too acidic or too basic, this can lead to a skin barrier problem, which can end up leading to skin disease. However, skin has an incredibly efficient buffering system to prevent this from happening. We know that cleansing the skin with soap increases the pH of the skin, which then returns to a more acidic pH within a few hours. But if you cleanse with

STRUCTURE OF THE STRATUM CORNEUM

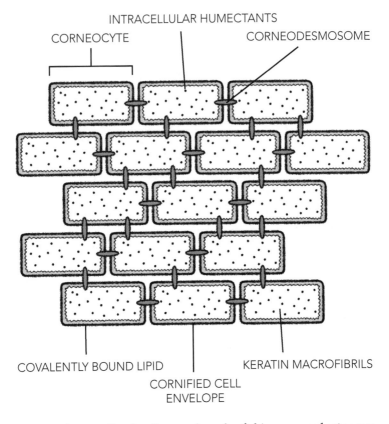

soap and immediately pile on a bunch of skincare products, you may cause more harm than good because your skin pH hasn't had time to recover. That's one reason why you may sometimes feel like your skin tingles or stings when you apply a skincare product right after cleansing – **the increased pH due to cleansing makes the skin more susceptible to irritation.**

Knowing a bit about how the stratum corneum functions can help you understand why dermatologists always tell you not to pick at spots or scratch itchy skin. The stratum corneum is home to small proteins that are responsible for stimulating your immune system to fight off intruders like bacteria. These small proteins are called 'cytokines' and they have names like interleukin-8, interleukin-6 and tumour necrosis factor alpha – terms you sometimes hear in reference to skin disease treatments. If fragments of the stratum corneum somehow make their way into the second layer of the skin (the dermis), this can cause inflammation to occur. Inflammation is the body's response to trauma or invasion and causes pain, redness and swelling of the area involved. If you have ever had a skin cyst rupture – like a sebaceous or epidermoid cyst or even an acne lesion – the stratum corneum fragments get into the dermis, release cytokines and a classic pimple, for example, occurs. Scratching itchy skin can also result in dislodging stratum corneum fragments into the skin, resulting in inflammation.

The fats of the stratum corneum

The fat layer – the lipid matrix – that embeds the corneocytes is made up of approximately 25 per cent cholesterol, 15 per cent free fatty acids and 50 per cent ceramides. In total, these make up 10 per cent of the weight of the stratum corneum and each type of fat is equally important to the way your skin functions.[9] It is important to know a bit about the science behind this fat layer because Big Skincare has started adding these fats to skincare products in order to market them as being great for 'skin barrier repair' or for 'helping to maintain a healthy skin barrier'. But how useful is it to apply these directly onto the skin? Should you be using a cream made of ceramides, for example? To answer that, we need to have a closer look at these fats.

We need to get technical for a moment: the spaces between the corneoctyes in the stratum corneum are filled with a lipid matrix that is referred to as a 'lamellar bilayer'. This is how all cell membranes are formed. You know that water and oil don't mix. Well, they don't mix in your body either! Fats are structured so that one end is afraid of water (hydrophobic) and the other is happy to be in water (hydrophilic). In a lipid bilayer, the ends that are happy to be in contact with water line up on either side, leaving the hydrophobic ends in the middle. Think of the lipid bilayer like a sandwich – the bread on either side is protecting the contents of the sandwich (your mayo-slathered tuna for example) from mixing with water. Basically, this way, your sandwich is 'waterproof'! The stratum corneum is actually waterproof in two directions – it generally does not want to let water in or out – and this unique two-way waterproofing is mainly due to the lipid bilayer.

SKINTELLIGENT TIP:

Using a ceramide-heavy moisturiser may do more harm than good

In recent years, the inclusion of ceramides in skincare products has become very trendy, but is the hype justified? Do you really need a skincare product specifically made with ceramides? This is a controversial area of skincare and research is still ongoing. Currently, there are 12 different subclasses of ceramides known, all of which have been identified in patients with atopic dermatitis, and an additional 6 subclasses found only in normal, healthy skin.[10] The names given to the different types of ceramides (and what you may read on an ingredient label of a ceramide-containing moisturiser) are based on the structure. The most abundant ceramide in the stratum corneum is CER-NP. Other ceramides that are thought to be essential for the normal functioning of the stratum corneum barrier are EOS, EODS, EOH and EOP.[11] **The bottom line with ceramides is that they may provide enhanced healing and moisturising to your skin *if you have atopic dermatitis (eczema)* but not if you have perfectly normal skin**; indeed, if you have normal skin, using a ceramide-heavy moisturiser may do more harm than good because it is important that in normal healthy skin all three types of fats exist in an equal ratio. Using a moisturiser that has an abundance of ceramides in it can 'unbalance' this ratio and affect how the skin barrier functions.

THE VIABLE EPIDERMIS

'Viable' means 'capable of living'. The viable epidermis is the part of the top layer of the skin sitting between the stratum corneum and the dermis. It is made up of a massive 70 per cent water. Though you don't often hear Big Skincare talk about the viable epidermis, it is where your skin pigment (colour) sits and it is responsible for creating the cells that make up the stratum corneum.

The lowest part of the viable epidermis is a single layer of cells called 'basal cells' or 'basal keratinocytes', which are stuck down to the basement membrane directly beneath it. The basement membrane is a thin layer of tissue that physically and functionally separates the epidermis from the dermis. Think of it as a sort of filter that allows certain amounts of water and cells to travel between the two. The boundary between the epidermis and dermis is undulating, meaning it is not just a straight line. This wave-like structure allows for more of the epidermis to come into contact with the dermis and lets the two interact, as they are dependent on each other to keep their normal structure and function.

The upper part of the dermis that is in contact with the epidermis is called the papillary dermis (papilla means 'projection' and refers to how at this level there are projections of the dermis into the epidermis). The lower part of the dermis not in contact with the epidermis is called the reticular dermis (reticular comes from the Latin word meaning 'net', because the reticular dermis tends to have denser collagen and elastin in it than the papillary dermis above it).

The basal keratinocytes can progress through three distinct phases as they make their way up to the top of the skin to be shed: the spinous phase, the granular phase and then, finally, the stratum corneum phase. The names of the phases relate to what the cells look like under a microscope at each stage of moving up through the epidermis.[12] The final step in the journey of a keratinocyte is called 'terminal differentiation' (which sounds rather ominous but is quite fitting) and this occurs at the junction between the granular layer and the stratum corneum. At this point, the 'viable' keratinocyte loses its nucleus (where the DNA is and what keeps the cell 'alive') and transforms into the flattened, 'dead' corneocyte filled with keratin filaments and water. And hence the stratum corneum is formed. **The entire epidermis is replaced every four weeks and the stratum corneum turnover time is about two weeks.**[13]

> *Keratinocyte*: the main cell of the epidermis that produces keratin, as well as the fats found between the cells and other important substances required for healthy skin.

When this normal progression of the basal cells through the epidermis is disrupted, skin problems occur. For example, psoriasis is a skin condition due to skin cell growth speeding up through the viable epidermis to the stratum corneum. Normal skin cells move through the epidermis and shed in about a month. In psoriasis, they do this in only 3–4 days and so don't shed when they get to the top. Instead, they pile up on the surface, resulting in the red plaques covered with scale, commonly seen on the back of the elbows, the front of the knees and the scalp.

The keratinocytes of the viable epidermis are little lipid and protein factories, and they function in a very controlled and regulated way to make everything the stratum corneum needs to function. When it comes to the epidermis, the stratum corneum is King (or Queen), so the entire viable epidermis is primarily geared towards getting the stratum corneum to function properly – think of the viable epidermis as a team of assistants. Like any great assistant, it is extremely responsive to changes in the stratum corneum. Any injury to the skin sets in motion a 'recovery' process to allow the barrier function of the stratum corneum to be restored within hours to days, depending on the age of the person and the severity of the injury.[14]

Skin stem cells

Some of the basal cells are in fact stem cells. Stem cells are often referred to as the body's 'raw materials' because they can multiply and generate various specialised cells that have different functions. Stem cells can also self-renew, meaning they basically live on forever. Stem cells in the basal layer of the epidermis allow the epidermis to keep on regenerating.[15] This is an intriguing idea when it comes to skincare – can skincare or supplements therefore somehow support these stem cells? You may think so considering the quantity of stem-cell-supporting or 'regenerating' products and supplements available on the market. However, **there is absolutely no scientific evidence that these skincare products or supplements have any positive impact on you or your skin**.

Melanocytes

Melanocytes are the pigment-producing cells of the epidermis, and they also live in the basal layer. There is one melanocyte for every ten basal keratinocytes in normal, sun-protected skin, but in areas that are heavily sun-damaged the ratio of melanocytes to basal keratinocytes can be one to one, which is one reason why, in heavily sun-damaged skin, you get spots of pigmentation known as 'solar lentigo' or 'sun freckles'.[16]

Melanocytes produce melanosomes, which are pigment-containing structures. Melanocytes are cells with long, winding arms (or tentacles) so that one melanocyte can be in contact with multiple keratinocytes throughout the viable epidermis. That's how melanosomes deposit melanin into keratinocytes, giving skin its colour. Lots of sun exposure stimulates melanocytes to make larger melanosomes (with more pigment in them). Within each keratinocyte, melanin forms a cap over the nucleus of the cell where it functions to protect the DNA within the nucleus from being damaged by sunlight. That's why the darker your skin is the lower your risk of developing skin cancer.

SKINTELLIGENT FACT:

Why humans have different skin colours

Every single human being in the world has the same number of melanocytes in their skin (1,000–2,000 melanocytes/mm^2 of skin – that's a lot of cells!).

The more melanin you have, the darker your skin colour and the more your skin absorbs UV (ultraviolet) radiation, specifically UVB. All humans originated from northern Africa 250,000 years ago. As humans moved north, where there is generally less sunshine, they required more UVB radiation to produce enough vitamin D in the skin, so they needed to produce less melanin to allow for that; in other words, as humans migrated north, they developed paler skin. It takes about 1,000 years for a migrant population to alter their melanocyte activity to allow for adequate skin protection and nutrient production.

Skin colour is not a reflection of education, values, money, beauty or intellect. It reflects what your melanocytes are programmed to do. It tells you what latitude your ancestors lived in for the 1,000 years before you were born. We must stand together in the face of racism and social injustice and support each other because we are all people, irrespective of the colour of our skin.

Problems with pigmentation are extremely common in people of all skin colours and 'pigment-correcting' cosmetic skincare products are a big moneymaker for Big Skincare. But **pigmentation problems are medical problems, not merely cosmetic issues**. Areas of skin can become lighter or darker than they should be naturally due to several reasons. In vitiligo, patches of skin completely lose their colour and become white ('depigmented') due to the destruction of the melanocytes. In albinism, in which people are born without skin colour at all and have very light skin, hair and eyes, the number of melanocytes is normal but they are unable to make fully pigmented melanosomes because of genetic defects in the enzymatic formation of melanin. On the other hand, the typical freckle is due to a localised increase in the production of pigment in a normal melanocyte, driven by sun exposure (that's why freckles fade when you aren't in the sun for a little while and appear again when you are) and partially by genetics. The darker a spot of pigmentation on the skin, the higher up in the epidermis the pigment is (so if you have a spot on your skin that looks black, but not blue, that means the melanin is in the stratum corneum). Regular skin moles – referred to as 'naevi' – are little groups ('nests') of melanocytes in the epidermis or dermis, or both, depending on the type of mole. They are genetic 'tumours' and are not sun-related.

As you can see, your epidermis is a complex powerhouse and is more than capable of looking after itself, even in the face of injury (thank goodness!). This should make you consider whether messing around with your epidermis through the use of cosmetic skincare, facials, microdermabrasion, microneedling or any other invasive or expensive treatment perhaps does more harm than good in the long run, if your skin is otherwise normal and healthy. I see the detrimental effects of the overuse of products and treatments on the skin every day in my clinical practice, which is why **I always advocate a 'less is more' approach when it comes to caring for your skin**!

HOW THE STRATUM CORNEUM IS MADE BY THE VIABLE EPIDERMIS

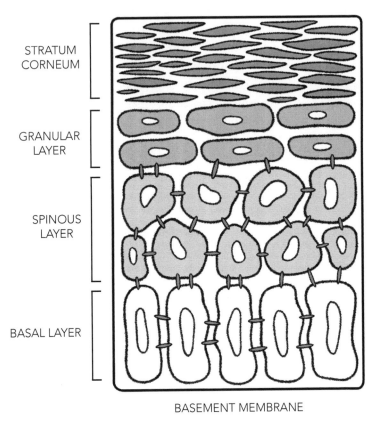

STRATUM CORNEUM

GRANULAR LAYER

SPINOUS LAYER

BASAL LAYER

BASEMENT MEMBRANE

THE DERMIS

Big Skincare pays a lot of attention to the dermis. We are constantly being told that the dermis thins as we age, resulting in wrinkles and sagging skin, creating a need for something that will 'rejuvenate', 'lift' or 'replenish' it from the outside in (or even from the inside in – hello collagen supplements!). But how true is this? What exactly is the dermis? How vital is it to keeping us looking good in our own skin? And, if it truly is that important, what do we really need to do to keep it from letting us down (no pun intended)?

Think of the dermis like a mattress and the fat underneath as the bed base (some people have a 'slimline' bed frame made of steel or wood, while other people have a chunkier 'divan'-type bed base – you get the idea). The dermis – your skin's mattress – is 3–5mm thick (for reference, a £1 coin is 3mm thick).

The main function of the dermis is to provide a tough mattress (or 'matrix') to support the many structures embedded in it, which include blood vessels, nerves, oil and sweat glands, and hairs. Collagen is the main fibre type making up the dermis and provides tensile strength (basically it prevents the skin from being torn by overstretching, like when you bend your knee). Mature collagen fibres are stronger than steel! Only 5 per cent of the dermis is elastin, though, which is the protein that allows the skin to be stretched in the first place, to allow your joints to move.

The most important cell in the dermis is the fibroblast and this cell makes all the components of the dermis – collagen, elastin and 'ground substance' (the jelly-like stuff that the collagen, elastin and fibroblasts live in). Ground substance is made up of glycosaminoglycans and glycoproteins, and makes up less than 2 per cent of the dry weight of the dermis. Its purpose is to function as lubrication for collagen fibres to slide past each other.

Hyaluronic acid

Hyaluronic acid (HA) is by far the most famous of the materials that make up the ground substance, but its true importance in skin function is questionable and certainly it is not anywhere near as important or useful as Big Skincare will make you believe it is when it comes to keeping your skin looking good.

HA does indeed have an extraordinary ability to hold

water – at least 1,000 times its dry weight – and it is often stated that HA is responsible for holding water in the dermis and maintaining its rigidity. But we also know that a decrease in HA in the dermis would almost certainly not be relevant to the signs of skin ageing like laxity and 'sag', as studies have shown that there is less TEWL in older versus younger people – the water content of older skin is not decreased.[17] **Topical products containing HA applied to the skin are unlikely to have any anti-ageing benefits** for this reason, but also because the molecule is too large to enter the dermis (see also pages 116 and 151).

Collagen

Collagen is produced by fibroblast cells. It starts out as individual strands or fibres called procollagen. Collagen is actually a bundle of individual procollagen fibres that have been 'cross-linked' (a type of very strong bond between two things) into a large, mature collagen fibre that is incredibly strong. In order for the procollagen fibres to cross-link into a large collagen fibre, they need to be exposed to an enzyme called prolyl hydroxylase and this enzyme can only work properly if ascorbic acid (vitamin C) is in the dermis too. This is why you so often hear Big Skincare go on and on about the idea of using topical vitamin C to 'aid' collagen production in the dermis. It also explains why nutritional deficiency in vitamin C results in blood vessel and skin fragility – a disease called scurvy. Without vitamin C, and therefore without the activity of prolyl hydroxylase, the cross-linked super strong collagen bundles will not form.

The rigidity of the dermis comes down to the collagen fibres. There are at least 15 genetically distinct types of collagen fibres in human skin, but collagen I comprises 90 per cent of the total collagen in skin.[18] (See page 52 for more on collagen.)

Sebaceous glands

Sebaceous glands are the oil-producing glands in the skin and they are incredibly important, not only for normal skin functioning but also for how skin looks. Selling you products that are 'oil-free' or in some other way reduce the amount of oil on your skin surface is a key goal of Big Skincare. But before we discuss some of the myths surrounding oily skin (see page 34), we need to first touch on how these glands work.

Sebaceous glands are attached to the upper part of the hair follicles and live in the dermis. Think of each sebaceous gland as an independent 'mini-organ' that is functionally and structurally related to the hair follicle. If the two were not attached, then common problems such as acne would not happen because sebum (oil) made by the sebaceous gland would be able to reach the skin's surface without obstruction (it's when oil and skin cells get stuck in the hair shaft leading out of the skin that acne pimples appear – see page 166). That's why we refer to problems like acne vulgaris as disorders of the 'pilosebaceous unit' – referring both to the hair follicle (pilus is Latin for 'hair') and the sebaceous gland together.

Sebaceous glands are always connected to hair follicles, except in some very specific situations. For example, if you look at the border of your lip, called the vermilion border, you may see some tiny little dots lining your lip. These are called Fordyce spots and are sebaceous glands that are not connected to hair follicles. In some people they are more noticeable than others, but don't try to squeeze them or get rid of them with creams because you can't!

Sebaceous gland cells called sebocytes are constantly multiplying, moving from the periphery of the duct to the centre of the duct as they mature, all the while accumulating lipid droplets. When they reach the end of their life cycle at the centre of the gland, they release their oil contents and the cell itself disintegrates. This process is controlled by multiple receptors sitting on the cells that respond to various signals generally coming from hormones, the most important of which is the androgen – a hormone responsible for growth and reproduction in men and to a lesser extent in women. Sebocytes can be hypersensitive to androgens in some people, leading to too much oil production. (More on this on pages 190–191.)

The number of sebaceous glands throughout the body varies tremendously; there are up to 900 glands/cm^2 on the face to fewer than 50 glands/cm^2 on the forearm. This is in direct relationship to the density of hair follicles on your body – you have more hair in terms of density (the hairs are closer together) on your head and your face than on your forearm, for example.

Hair follicles

The hair follicle is the structure from which your hairs grow and has three parts:

1. The infundibulum: the skin surface to the opening of the sebaceous gland.
2. The isthmus: from the sebaceous gland to the arrector pili muscle (the tiny muscle that contracts to make the hair stand up straight in the skin and gives you 'goosebumps' when you feel cold!).
3. The inferior segment: from the arrector pili muscle to the base of the hair follicle.

At the base of the hair follicle sits the dermal papilla, which is the command centre for that individual hair and is the part of the follicle that receives the blood supply and nutrients necessary for hair growth. The hair shaft is the part of the hair follicle that you see as hair, sticking out of the skin. The hair follicle is an extremely relevant structure to skin disease because, when the cells of the follicle don't work the way they should, this leads to skin diseases like acne vulgaris.

SUBCUTANEOUS TISSUE

A description of how skin works would not be complete without mentioning the subcutaneous tissue – the layer of fat directly beneath the dermis. This fat works as a shock absorber, is a high-calorie storage area for energy and also helps with regulating body temperature. From a practical point of view, when it comes to how our skin looks, it is relevant because the fat layer shrinks as we get older, especially in sun-exposed sites like the backs of the hands and the face. This loss of fat (fat atrophy) is one of the major contributors to the 'ageing' face, along with resorption or thinning of the bones of the face.

AN OVERVIEW OF SKIN ANATOMY

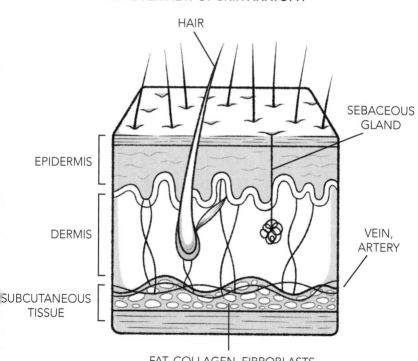

HAIR

SEBACEOUS GLAND

EPIDERMIS

DERMIS

VEIN, ARTERY

SUBCUTANEOUS TISSUE

FAT, COLLAGEN, FIBROBLASTS

Key definitions

- The *keratinocyte* is the cell of the epidermis that produces keratin.
- The *corneocyte* is a flattened keratinocyte that has lost its nucleus and sits at the top of the skin, in the stratum corneum layer of the epidermis.
- *Keratin* is a protein – your hair and nails are made of keratin.
- *Keratinisation* is the process of keratinocytes becoming corneocytes.
- *Natural moisturising factors (NMFs)* are substances, usually small proteins, within the corneocytes that are hygroscopic so have the ability to absorb and hold water from the air in the cell.
- *Transepidermal water loss (TEWL)* is the amount of water that passively evaporates through skin to the external environment.
- A *humectant* is a substance that promotes the retention of water (it attracts and holds water).
- *Ceramides* are a type of fat (lipid) that make up 50 per cent of the fats in the top layer of the skin.

2

The Myth of the Skin 'Type'

What's your skin type? If you are reading this book, I am fairly certain you have pondered this question or someone trying to sell you something has asked you this. The standard categories of skin 'types' are dry, oily, sensitive and combination, but Big Skincare has invented these to more easily guide you to purchase specific products, supposedly 'made' for your skin type.

In trying to make purchasing products easier, Big Skincare has created a whole lot of confusion for you, the consumer, because, in fact, **there is no such thing as a skin 'type'**. Skin is skin – it can't be categorised into a 'type' based on how it feels to you. What you experience are called 'symptoms'. That's one way I assess a patient's skin – by asking them what their symptoms are. They may say 'dry', 'tight', 'oily', 'itchy', 'stingy' or 'sore' – and this is usually in relation to the use of a product or treatment or an underlying skin problem that needs to be corrected.

> **The bottom line**: Fundamentally, all skin is 'combination' skin – everyone has more oil in the T zone (the nose, mid-forehead and chin) compared to the rest of the face.

If your skin is excessively oily, dry or sensitive, this is a reaction to something; it isn't normal skin. Figuring out what is causing that problem and then helping you find a suitable solution is my goal with this book.

SKINTELLIGENT FACT:

The real skin types

In my daily practice, the only time I refer to a skin 'type' is when I am examining a patient for skin cancer and I need to document their skin 'phototype', which is a way to classify skin based on how it reacts when exposed to sunlight (tanning versus burning), from I to VI – known as the Fitzpatrick skin type.[1] Skin type I always burns and never tans and is someone with very pale white skin, blue or green eyes and blonde or red hair, while skin type VI never burns and tans very darkly, with dark brown or black skin. You are born with a skin type and it does not change during your lifetime.

OILY SKIN

One of the most common complaints I see in my patients is excessively oily skin, starting with teenagers, who usually also have spots, all the way to adult men and women who have perfectly clear skin but develop excess oil production in their teens that persists into adulthood (for some men) or after having children or around the menopause (for women).

There are two sources of oil (also referred to as lipid or sebum) in the skin: the sebaceous glands that live in the reticular (lower) dermis in association with hair follicles to form pilosebaceous units and secrete sebum onto the surface of the skin (see page 198), and the lipid layer in the stratum corneum (between the corneocytes – see page 18). In adults, the lipids found in the stratum corneum contribute only 3–6 per cent of the total surface lipids of the skin.[2] This is important to know because not all oil on (or in) the skin is the same or serves the same purpose. **Using skincare to remove one 'type' of oil from the skin can often result in removing the other one as well, leading to skin problems.**

In adults, the amount of oil on the forehead varies between 150 and 300ug of lipid/cm^2. When there is too much oil on the skin, this is generally due to having too many sebaceous glands in terms of volume and size (so bigger sebaceous glands than what would be considered 'normal' or necessary).[3] Having oily skin can be a cosmetic nuisance (make-up just doesn't sit right and the skin is shiny, but not in the healthy 'dewy' way we want it to be), but it can also predispose to getting acne vulgaris (see Chapter 12) and sebaceous hyperplasia (see page 38), as well as the overuse of drying skincare products.

A widely held belief is that if you 'strip' the surface of the skin of oil (with lots of cleansing or the use of alcohol-based 'toners') and make it dry, this will stimulate the glands to produce even more oil. In biology, this is called a 'negative feedback loop' and is how many systems in our bodies maintain tight control of how our systems function. This notion about skin surface oil is so widely believed that even some seemingly well-respected online resources propagate this idea.[4]

From a common-sense, first-principle point of view, this notion is completely illogical: for a negative feedback loop to exist, there must be some type of signal by which the sebaceous gland can 'detect' that there is more or less oil on the skin surface. In 1958, pioneering dermatologists proved that this was not the case by performing a series of incredibly simple yet ingenious experiments on the foreheads of what they referred to as 'sebaceous athletes' – 125 inmates in a Philadelphia prison who produced above-average amounts of oil.[5] Though I do not condone the ethics of this type of research (these clinical experiments would never be allowed today), it has given us some extraordinary insights into how skin works. In direct contradiction to the feedback theory is this: *the sebaceous gland functions continuously, without regard to what is on the surface of the skin.*

What about the theory that the more often you remove the oil from your face, the more seems to appear? Let's say you wipe off the surface oil from your forehead every 30 minutes – you may find you wipe more off every 30 minutes than you do if you were to wipe only once every 3 hours. Is that possible? Are you stimulating more oil to be secreted by the glands each time you remove the surface oil?

No – but there is a good explanation for why it feels that way. There is always preformed sebum sitting in your oil glands ready and waiting to flow out onto your skin's surface at a constant rate. When you remove or wipe off the surface oil, you remove some from the tunnels between the cells as well. When the surface oil is removed, the stored fat in the gland immediately flows to the surface filling in the tunnels between the cells and coming onto the skin surface, giving the appearance of a more rapid rate of secretion initially. It takes 2–3 hours for your baseline level of surface oil to reaccumulate.

So, sebum production on the skin surface is a continuous process in which the rate of generation of the cells and their loss is in 'equilibrium'. The amount of oil that can be delivered to the skin surface at any one time per unit area of skin is directly proportional to the total number and size of the sebaceous glands; the larger the glands, the more sebum is produced in a given time.

Why is it, then, that skin dryness can make you feel like you are temporarily less oily? Some topical treatments used for acne can be irritating to the sweat glands that are in your skin and temporarily cause less sweat to be produced. The other thing that can happen is that increased scaliness due to irritation or dryness of the stratum corneum can increase the sebum-holding capacity of the tunnels between the cells of the stratum corneum or even temporarily 'block' the hair follicle opening onto the surface of the skin, so less oil flows onto the surface of the skin.

SKINTELLIGENT FACT:

Why your face feels oilier when you sweat

Good news! Sweating does not stimulate your sebaceous glands to produce more oil. An increase in
temperature aids the flow of preformed stored sebum
to the surface of the skin. Remember also that the presence of sweat gives the appearance of oiliness – if some
oil is on your skin, even a little bit of sweat will go a long
way in creating the appearance of oily skin. That is why
people with oily skin find their oiliness is less of a problem in the winter and more of a problem in hot, humid
climates – the difference is due to the amount of water
on the skin.

If you feel you have too much oil on your skin, you may find
yourself asking the question why we have oil on our skin in the
first place, as it can be such a cosmetic nuisance. Well, skin surface oil actually plays several important roles in keeping skin
healthy and makes up part of the 'skin barrier' function. It does
this in three ways: it tends to repel water; it provides antioxidants to the skin surface; and it is antibacterial. Mixed in with the
sebum that comes onto your skin surface are the antioxidants
vitamin E and coenzyme Q10. These help protect your skin from
damage from UV light (sunlight), pollution and mechanical and
chemical insults. Sebum is also strongly antibacterial to most
bacteria and to *candida albicans* (a type of fungal disease).

The bottom line: If you find that you are generally very oily,
this is a sign that you truly have an increased amount of oil in
your skin, but if you find that occasionally you are suddenly
oilier, this is more likely due to sweating.

SKINTELLIGENT TIP:

When you can see oil glands in your skin and what to do about it

'Sebaceous hyperplasia' are super common little bumps on excessively oily skin, but you may never have heard of them because they can't be treated with lotions or potions. They are small - 2-6mm in diameter - cream-coloured little bumps that have a classic appearance under the dermatoscope (the handheld magnifying device dermatologists use to examine skin): they have yellow globules of sebum surrounding a central crater and often a ring of telangiectasia (dilated capillaries - see page 210) around them. Sebaceous hyperplasia tend to occur on areas of the face that have a lot of densely packed oil glands, like the nose, forehead, chin and cheeks. 'Hyperplasia' means enlargement of an organ or tissue. In this case, it's the single oil gland that gets enlarged and becomes prominent and visible. Treatment involves physical destruction of the spot, with electrosurgery, laser or a shallow shave.

DRY SKIN

Dry skin is the visible result of a defective stratum corneum – the very top layer of the skin (see page 14). When the stratum corneum doesn't work the way it should, there is increased transepidermal water loss (TEWL – see page 15) and a decreased ability of the stratum corneum to take up and retain sufficient water to maintain a soft, supple, resilient, smooth top of the skin. When the stratum corneum is 'dry' and its structure is damaged, it can no longer carry out its multiple and diverse protective functions.

But dry skin isn't just one thing; it should be thought of as a variety of skin reactions ranging in severity from a sensation of mild tightness in the skin through to flaking and scaling all the way to skin damage and even infection. The hallmark of this more severe end of dry skin is redness and itchiness – what we call 'eczema' or 'atopic dermatitis' (see Chapter 14). Dry skin can also make your skin look dull because it doesn't reflect light well.

SKINTELLIGENT FACT:

Dry skin is not the opposite of oily skin

If dry skin were the opposite of oily skin, you would expect that in skin diseases characterised by dry skin (like eczema) the skin would have little sebum secretion; however, we know that this is not the case and that in the majority of dry skin conditions sebum secretion is within the normal range.[6] Dry or non-dry skin is in reference to the water content of the skin, not the oil content or the amount of surface oil.

All different types of dry skin can be caused by both external and internal factors. External factors that lead to the appearance of dry skin include the use of chemicals for cleansing, environmental pollutants, chemical pollutants encountering the skin such as certain fragrances, preservatives and botanicals, some topical medical treatments, as well as the level of humidity in the air and exposure to sunlight. Internal factors include such diverse things as the age and mental state of the person as well as raised cortisol levels due to stress or sleep deprivation.[7]

SKINTELLIGENT TIP:

You can't hydrate your skin by drinking lots of water

One of the most common things I hear from patients is that they drink lots of water every day, but they still suffer from dry or irritated skin or acne. Adequate skin hydration is, of course, critical for maintaining skin health, but can you really hydrate your skin by drinking lots of water?

One study looked at just this and concluded that drinking water or fluids in excess of 'normal' intake is unnecessary; it doesn't add to skin hydration, treat acne or just generally lead to 'healthier' skin.[8] The only exception to this is people who are medically unwell. Skin 'turgor' is the medical term for skin elasticity. Normally, hydrated skin should bounce back into place within a second or two. If your skin turgor is poor, it means it takes longer for your skin to return to its usual position. In medicine, we use skin turgor as a crude clinical sign of dehydration. In healthy individuals outside of an intensive care unit, hydration status is generally not something you can assess via the skin. I'm afraid **the saying 'drink more water to get plump, hydrated skin' is nothing but an old wives' tale.**

Flaky skin and dry skin are the same thing – when your skin gets dry, it gets a bit flaky. The two terms can be used interchangeably. Dry skin is abnormal skin shedding, or 'desquamation', due to a diverse number of underlying causes. In dermatology speak, it is a 'cutaneous reaction pattern', meaning it is a skin response to something else going on; it is a symptom of a problem, not the problem itself.

The corneocytes normally shed off the top of your skin in small groups, small enough that they are not visible on the skin surface to the naked eye (see page 15). But when this process of shedding is disturbed in any way, the corneocytes collect in visible clumps – what you see as 'scales' – and this produces a rough skin texture and appearance.[9]

Sebaceous gland secretions (the sebum or oil that sits on your skin's surface) play an insignificant part in keeping your skin flake-free and 'hydrated'. This can be seen best in children before they hit puberty; they have essentially no sebum production at all but still manage to have smooth, well-hydrated skin and no problems with dryness or flakiness. And most kids under the age of 12 have never used a facial moisturiser!

SKINTELLIGENT TIP:

Don't waste your money on skincare products claiming to have 'natural moisturising factors' in them

Natural moisturising factors (NMFs) are small molecules that act as 'humectants', which means they directly pull in water (see page 72). There are some skincare brands that make products with NMFs in them claiming they can work to hydrate skin.

However, NMFs in the skin are confined to the corneocyte; virtually all the free water in the stratum corneum is inside the corneoctyes. The corneocyte doesn't let anything aside from water and a few specific molecules enter and leave the cell via specialised 'tunnels' called aquaporins (there are specific ones for urea and water, for example).

These NMFs work *in the cell* as humectants in order to maintain corneocyte, and therefore stratum corneum, hydration levels. They cannot enter the cell when you apply them to the skin (unless there is a specific aqua-porin for the molecule). **It makes absolutely zero basic science sense to say that you can apply NMFs to the skin and they will somehow magically increase skin hydration. They don't. They won't.**

Just another example of the pseudoscience market-ing that Big Skincare propagates to look 'scientific' and sell you products. Please don't waste your time or money using skincare products containing NMFs.

The bottom line: Dry skin itself isn't a medical concern unless it becomes sore, itchy or inflamed.

SENSITIVE (REACTIVE) SKIN

The term 'sensitive skin' is used by many people to refer to their skin 'type'. However, and perhaps surprising to many, 'sensitive skin' as a skin condition or a set of symptoms is very difficult to define and diagnose. Whether or not 'sensitive skin' is a true skin condition is controversial, but there have been, in recent years, some suggestions of how we can define it clin-ically: 'sensitive skin' is characterised by abnormal stinging, burning and tingling sensations (and sometimes pain or itch-ing) in response to multiple factors that may be physical, chemical, psychological or hormonal. Redness of the skin is often but not always a feature. However, there is no way to test for this condition; it is diagnosed purely based on medical history.

It is important to realise that what causes these symptoms (the 'pathophysiology') collectively known as 'sensitive skin' is not known – we don't know why certain people react to certain things the way they do. What we do know is that it is not immunologic or allergic and there are no abnormal changes in the structure of the skin (histological abnormalities) seen in skin samples (biopsies) taken from patients who report having 'sensitive skin'.[10]

What could be happening in these patients is that their 'skin tolerance threshold' is low, potentially due to impaired barrier function, which leads to too much TEWL. This in turn leads to dryness and disruption of the top layer of the skin, which can allow irritants to then enter the skin and stimulate an inflammatory response. The term 'reactive' skin is probably better than sensitive skin. And it is super common – I see it in my clinic every day, and in Europe over 50 per cent of individuals report having reactive skin.[11] The prevalence seems to be mostly related to environmental factors and increases in the summer, suggesting that UV exposure has a role.

SKINTELLIGENT TIP:

There's no need to avoid fragrance in skincare

I'm often asked whether you need to avoid fragrance in skincare. And the answer is simply, not if you are not allergic or sensitive to it. Fragrances are one of the most common causes of allergic contact allergy to skincare products, but most people are fine with them. The same goes for essential oils. If you like using these types of products, then go for it.

If you think you are suffering from 'reactive skin', have a look at the products you are using and try to cut down to only the absolute bare minimum – for most people, that is a cleanser at night, a moisturiser and perhaps some sunscreen. Excess use of skincare disrupts your skin's natural barrier function and can lead to a whole host of problems, including what you might describe as 'sensitive skin'. If you have a skin condition or problem, see a consultant dermatologist and get the right diagnosis and treatment (or keep reading this book and hopefully some of your questions will be answered!). (See page 277 for how to find the right dermatologist for you.)

EVERYONE'S SKIN IS FUNDAMENTALLY THE SAME

I can hear your screams of protest to this statement already, but just hear me out . . .

The basic structure of everyone's skin is the same – otherwise these two chapters you have just read would be pointless. However, just like some people have diabetes mellitus and others have dodgy knees, lots of people have a huge variety of skin problems. The more accurate thing to say is: **everyone has different skin problems, different personal preferences and different expectations of treatments and products**. Some people don't have any skin problems at all (or they don't really care either way and that's totally fine). And if a moisturiser 'works' for one person but doesn't for another, it's because they have differing skin problems that require different management, different personal preferences or different expectations for that moisturiser. But it's not because their basic skin structure is different; every human has a dermis and an epidermis composed of the same types of cells and molecules.

And that completes your introduction to the most general types of symptoms you can experience with your skin: oiliness, dryness and sensitivity. Most of us will experience all three of these issues at some point in our lives, and will almost certainly try at least one or two cosmetic skincare products to tackle them. Unfortunately, often these attempts don't help the situation or can even make it worse. See Part 2 for a deep dive into how skincare works (or doesn't), but first let's address the controversial topic of skin ageing.

3

How Skin Changes as We Age

Understanding what happens to skin as we age is fundamental to being able to 'manage' it or try to 'prevent' it in an intelligent way (though the idea that you can 'prevent' your skin from ageing is very controversial – the ageing process is inevitable, unfortunately). Big Skincare is focused on selling you the next best device/lotion/food supplement/random product that will either prevent your skin from ageing at all or will turn back the hands of time. But do any of these bazillion products actually do anything helpful?

Ageing, or the passage of time, affects human beings from the inside out – we refer to this as 'intrinsic' ageing; it cannot be stopped, it just happens to us all, to some perhaps more than others, and in some more quickly than others. But it happens. With skin, intrinsic ageing manifests in how the skin functions and what it looks like, and is very different to extrinsic ageing – that which is caused by forces outside of us. The main cause of extrinsic ageing is sunlight – I would suggest that sunlight accounts for over 95 per cent of what we think of as 'extrinsic' ageing. Understanding how skin responds differently to intrinsic and extrinsic ageing can help us figure out how to delay or even reverse some of those changes.

Intrinsic ageing causes a decrease in the actual cells of both the epidermis and the dermis, along with a gradual reduction in the amount of collagen and elastin that gives the dermis its structure and volume. Extrinsic ageing is mainly due to exposure to UV light (referred to as 'photoageing'), as well as cigarette smoking in those who smoke, and this causes abnormal elastin molecules to get deposited into the papillary (upper) dermis as well as low-level chronic inflammation leading to thickening of the epidermis.

You therefore have both abnormal thinning and abnormal thickening of the skin happening at the same time, leading to the appearance of ageing skin – fine and coarse wrinkles, pigmentation, thread veins (telangiectasia) and skin sagging (though this is mainly due to changes in the muscles and bone structure of the face).

In clinical practice, we see two different presentations of skin ageing: people with darker skin get 'hypertrophic' skin ageing with leathery skin, coarse wrinkles and pigmentation changes, while fair-skinned people get 'atrophic' changes with the appearance of thread veins (telangiectasia), finer lines and enlarged pores.

SKINTELLIGENT TIP:

The butt skin test

I get a lot of patients who are sceptical about the importance of sunshine avoidance to keep their skin looking young and healthy. It is easy to think that photoageing represents just an 'acceleration' of normal (intrinsic) ageing, but this is not the case. To make my point I have come up with what I call 'The Butt Skin Test'.

The closest skin on your body to your normal or 'perfect' non-sun-damaged, non-photodamaged skin is your butt skin. Yup – the skin on your bum. I look at bum skin every day (that is not as weird as it sounds – it's part of a full skin check when I am examining people to look for skin cancer) and I know that generally bum skin is your best skin. And your bum skin has probably never been subjected to a facial or a hyaluronic acid serum or even a moisturiser (who moisturises their bum?). And it looks pretty awesome (the skin, that is!). Unless you have used tons of sunbeds naked for a long time or you regularly sunbathe in your birthday suit, your bum displays your best skin. A close second is the skin on the underside of your forearm. Isn't that beautiful skin? If you are older, then it might be a little bit crêpey or wrinkled, but it should be unblemished and smooth. The bum skin of older people is also generally slightly loose and a little bit wrinkled because of gravity and general intrinsic ageing of the collagen and elastin in the dermis, but the skin surface itself should be in great, unblemished condition.

What we associate with young skin – plumpness, fullness, elastic resilience – cannot be explained away with simple statements like 'your skin gets drier as you age'. We have to look a little more deeply into the complexity of the architecture and structures in the skin to understand how and why skin changes as we age.

HOW THE EPIDERMIS AGES

I like to use the word 'specious' when talking about skin ageing. 'Specious' means something is superficially or logically possible or plausible, but actually wrong. This happens a lot with skin. Because it is highly visible, it is easy to see how this can happen.

One specious 'universal truth' is that as we age the epidermis becomes thinner, especially in areas of chronic sun exposure. The truth is that chronic sun exposure thickens the epidermis because chronic damage to the skin generally stimulates a protective response, one of which is thickening of the layers of cells (known as hyperplasia). If non-exposed skin is looked at under a microscope (a skin biopsy), the epidermis looks thinner in older people because the lower surface of the epidermis loses its undulating contour – basically, it gets flatter looking and there is less surface area contact between the epidermis and dermis (which is, coincidentally, why older skin is more susceptible to being torn easily). The flattening of the epidermis also means that there are fewer basal cells per unit surface area, and this decreases the number of new skin cells (keratinocytes) being produced – which is partially why older people have drier skin. The new cells are also differently shaped compared to those of younger skin – rather than being perfectly shaped, the ones made in older skin are a bit more randomly shaped and, when it comes to cells, shape affects function.

There are two widely held explanations for why skin gets dry-looking as we age. The first is that there is excessive loss of water through a defective stratum corneum because the stratum corneum itself is unable to hold water properly and therefore becomes dry and brittle. The second reason is that the water content of the dermis is too low to provide moisture to the epidermis above it. Both of these explanations are incorrect. When transepidermal water loss (TEWL – see page 15) is measured in both young and old people, there is less TEWL in the older subjects.[1] In fact, the stratum corneum is not thinner in older people, with a fully competent barrier function. Generally, the rate of TEWL does not change during the ageing process.

The difference that ageing brings is the ability of the stratum corneum to *recover* once it has been damaged.[2] **Younger people generally recover faster from things like hangovers and the flu – the same applies to the stratum corneum.**

There are several theories that could explain why this happens. The production of new keratinocytes in the viable epidermis slows down and the number of structural proteins needed for the corneocyte envelopes to form well (like filaggrin) also seems to decline with age. Other things slow down as well – like the production of the fats between the cells in the stratum corneum. Remember that the different fats are made by the skin cells, so if the production of those is slowed down, then less fat is formed, and these fats are super important to keep the stratum corneum functioning normally (see page 19). Some studies have shown that the aged stratum corneum has more than a 30 per cent reduction in total lipid content compared to a young stratum corneum.[3] This is due primarily to reduced cholesterol synthesis and levels of cholesterol in the lipid matrix, while levels of ceramides seemed to stay fairly consistent.

A key point here is that the cholesterol in your skin is made in the same way as it is in your liver, through the action of an enzyme called HMG-CoA reductase. This enzyme is blocked by a group of medicines called statins, which are almost universally prescribed to people over the age of 55 to lower cholesterol, as part of the primary prevention of heart attacks and heart disease. Statins are inhibitors of HMG-CoA reductase and that's how they work to lower cholesterol. But this will also affect how well the skin can make cholesterol, which directly affects the structure and function of the stratum corneum. In this way, statins are often a contributor to the dry, itchy skin seen in older people or those who take statins.[4] If you take a statin and are also suffering with dry, itchy skin, you may want to talk to your doctor about whether it could be affecting your skin.

Older skin has a slightly higher skin surface pH than younger skin, which can also be one of the factors contributing to its delay in recovery. In addition, when the barrier is disrupted, for example by scratching the skin, the delay in recovery opens a theoretical 'window' for things to infiltrate the skin and lead to inflammation and itchiness. This can further predispose older skin to developing atopic and contact dermatitis.

HOW THE DERMIS AGES

Collagen

Collagen makes up more than 90 per cent of the dry weight of human skin. It plays a central role in virtually all anti-ageing and skin rejuvenation treatments touted by Big Skincare. But what actually is collagen, what does it do for skin and – perhaps most importantly – can it be manipulated to reverse the effects of ageing?

As we age, the collagen in our dermis becomes stiffer and more resistant to being broken down. This is a bit of an odd finding because we generally think of old skin as loose and saggy. So, what is going on here? In simple terms, healthy young collagen is arranged in a neat, tidy network in the dermis, but as we age this network becomes disorganised and messy – resulting in decreased skin tension and changes in the way the skin looks. Let me explain this with a little more detail . . .

The most abundant type of collagen in the dermis is collagen I. The collagen in your skin is constantly but slowly being 'turned over', meaning old collagen is being broken down and replaced by new collagen. But this breakdown and replacement of mature collagen is extremely slow and there are only four enzymes made by humans that can actually do it! These enzymes are called 'collagenases' and are part of a 'family' of enzymes called matrix metalloproteinases (MMPs). Of the four enzymes that can break down collagen, only one of them (known as MMP-1) is responsible for normal collagen turnover in the skin. So there isn't a lot of collagen being broken down and replaced on a regular basis.

Of course, your skin wants to preserve its collagen, so you also have natural inhibitors of MMPs in your skin called 'tissue inhibitors of matrix metalloproteinases' (TIMPS) and they work hard to slow down collagen breakdown. The type 1 collagen in your skin is mega stable and it can take about 30 years for it to be replaced!

However, this is a double-edged sword for your skin: the slow turnover of collagen I allows for damaged collagen (due to age or photodamage, for example) to form cross-links in your normal healthy collagen. As they cannot be efficiently broken down or removed entirely due to the slow MMP activity, you start to accumulate fragmented collagen fibres within the dermis as you age and this leads to changes in how your skin looks – it becomes less 'bouncy', with less resilience. Below you can see the neatly arranged collagen fibres in younger skin and the disorganised collagen fibres in older skin.

The bottom line: The accumulation of fragmented collagen is a key reason why our skin changes appearance as we age.[5]

DERMIS OF YOUNG VERSUS OLD

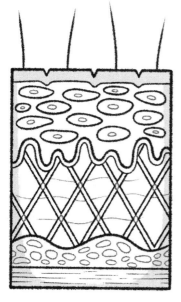

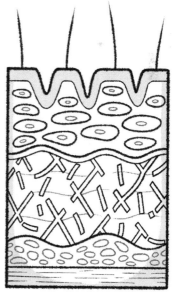

YOUNGER SKIN   OLDER SKIN

New collagen is made when the skin is physically damaged, such as in an accident if you get a cut or in surgery when your skin is cut – this is called 'neocollagenesis'. Whenever skin is cut and then heals, a scar is formed, and a scar is actually new collagen that is made by fibroblasts in response to the injury. However, this new collagen starts out as collagen III, which is a lot stiffer than collagen I. We refer to collagen III as being 'fibrous' and, when these fibrous collagen fibres are produced in the dermis, it results in stiff, rigid skin that looks different from your normal skin – we call this a scar.[6] In keloid scars (thick, raised scars that are bigger than the original wound), collagen III is initially formed, but is then replaced by collagen I in a disorganised arrangement, resulting in the thickened, raised skin you see with a keloid scar. Hypertrophic scars are similar to keloid scars (but are the same size as the original wound) with increased collagen deposition, but the collagen is more organised.[7]

Neocollagenesis is triggered by anything that damages the dermis – and this includes when the damage is inflicted on purpose like in some types of anti-ageing treatments (more on this in Part 5). But a key point to remember is that injury stimulates the production of collagen III first, before it undergoes changes to become collagen I.

So how are the fibroblasts involved in all this? Think of the fibroblast like a trampoline, and the metal loops and cables pulling it taut are the collagen fibres. On the surface of the fibroblast (the trampoline) there are little attachment sites called integrins. The collagen fibres are connected to the integrins and via the integrins pull the fibroblast taut. This stretch is required for the fibroblast to produce normal levels of collagen and MMPs. This is what happens in young, healthy, non-sun-exposed skin. In photodamaged or aged skin, the integrins no longer attach the fibroblast to the collagen fibres and the fragmented collagen fibres are unable to provide any traction on the integrins. Without the loops (integrins) or the ropes (collagen fibres), the trampoline (fibroblast) collapses.

The reduced collagen production and increased collagen fragmentation further reduces the mechanical tension and so you get continued loss of collagen. Once the ropes holding the trampoline taut are weakened or broken, it can be very difficult to get it taut again. It is important here to note that UV radiation (sunlight) stimulates collagen-degrading MMP activity and suppresses collagen production.

A key interesting fact is that fibroblasts don't seem to get old. When comparing fibroblasts from severely photodamaged forearm skin to matched protected skin, collagen and

COLLAPSED VERSUS STRETCHED FIBROBLAST

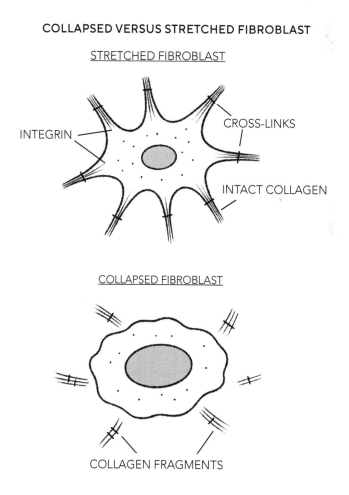

STRETCHED FIBROBLAST

INTEGRIN

CROSS-LINKS

INTACT COLLAGEN

COLLAPSED FIBROBLAST

COLLAGEN FRAGMENTS

MMP-1 production was the same.[8] Fibroblasts examined from sun-protected skin of individuals over 80 years old compared to those from skin of individuals under 30 showed only a very small decrease in the cell's ability to produce collagen. This supports the idea that the **real cause of the appearance of aged skin is the fragmented collagen itself**.

The dermis definitely thins in old age – there is less collagen per surface area, and it is less dense.[9] The thickness of the dermis increases significantly up until the age of 50 – the reticular (lower) dermis is initially 1.6mm thick in the first months of life to a maximum of 3.2mm at 50 years old, with a doubling of the thickness of the collagen bundles, and then it thins out to about 1.3mm in those who are 95 years old. That's quite a substantial change. Surprisingly, from the age of ten, the number of fibroblasts in the dermis stays constant at around 2,000 cells/mm^2.[10]

Men have a thicker dermis than women, which may partly explain why women tend to look older more quickly than men.

Elastin

In protected skin, the changes in elastin as we age are different in the top and bottom of the dermis. In the papillary (upper) dermis, there is a loss in the number of elastic fibres and the remaining ones are no longer in the neat configuration they were in younger skin (similar to what happens with collagen, which becomes disorganised, as we saw above). This change is the explanation for why older unexposed skin develops a finely wrinkled surface (again, bum skin is a good example of this). In the reticular (lower) dermis, the elastin fibres actually become thicker, more numerous, more branched and disarrayed. This elastin is structurally abnormal and the result is a loss of resiliency when it is stretched. These changes start from as early as 30 years old!

WHAT CAUSES FACIAL SKIN SAGGING AS WE AGE?

There are two theories – both valid – to explain why facial skin sags with age (think jowls, lack of a defined jawline and a deepened nasolabial fold – the line between your cheek and your upper lip).

The first theory is that gravity is to blame, combined with the weakening of the ligaments that anchor the dermis to the bone structure of the face.[11] The weakening of these ligaments is due to repeated muscle activity during facial expression. However, this concept was called into question in a long-term study that suggested that the vertical descent of facial skin and tissue was not the major component of ageing skin.[12]

The other theory is that skin sagging is due to volume change. A group of researchers dissected 40 cadavers and found a dramatic decrease in the amount of facial fat in the group of cadavers over 75 years old. This loss of fat is the main cause of volume loss as we age. Along with the effects of gravity, these are the underlying problems that lead to sagging skin, and therefore the visible signs of an ageing face.[13]

The major skin aspect related to skin sagging that changes as we age is elastic recovery (due to the changes we see in elastin resiliency, as described above); in other words, the skin's ability to 'bounce back' from being stretched (think of a new pair of leggings versus a pair you have worn and washed 100 times – the old pair sags a bit at the knees and the bum). The combination of the loss of fat in the face combined with skin that has been stretched and lost its elasticity leads to the appearance of 'sagging skin', along with the effects of gravity and weakening of the facial ligaments.

The only way to break through the noise of the Big Skincare marketing machine is to understand how skin ages – both inside and out. The unique thing about skin ageing is that you can see it happening – the signs are very clear. This is both a help and a hindrance; you can take action when you see something happening to try to delay or even prevent it, but seeing things changing, even gradually, can also profoundly affect your well-being and self-confidence.

However, now that you understand why or how something is happening to your skin, I hope you feel empowered to both accept that your skin changes with time, and also seek out the most potentially effective (and cost-effective!) treatments while maintaining realistic expectations for what is or is not achievable. Let's now take a critical look at skincare products and ingredients so you can start making more 'skintelligent' decisions about what you actually want to put on your skin every day.

PART 2

How Skincare Works (Or Doesn't)

Patients should be told that it may just be the act of consistently following a skincare regime that has an effect, not the act of consistently following a particular skincare regimen.

Lionel Bercovitch and Clifford Perlis in
Dermatoethics[1]

Modern skincare wasn't invented by doctors. It wasn't invented by scientists or chemists either. It was (and, for the most part, still is) the concept of a handful of savvy entrepreneurs who were (and are) keen to exploit the vanity and insecurities of women and men.

The fabrication of modern 'beauty products' as an industry began in the early twentieth century, when Helena Rubinstein (original name Chaja, born in Krakow, Poland in 1870) arrived in New York in 1914. She had made her way to the United States via Melbourne, having escaped from her parents in Poland who wanted her to marry a wealthy local widower. While in Melbourne, she had started selling a face cream called Crème Valaze – apparently invented by a Dr Jacob Lykusky in Krakow. However, historical research has failed to identify this

doctor or anyone with that name working as a medical professional at the time. More than likely this was all part of one of
Rubinstein's (many) clever marketing schemes. In all probabil-
ity she had created the cream herself – a mix of lanolin, soft
paraffin, distilled water and pine bark extract. Pine bark extract
is purported to be an antioxidant and was meant to repair connective tissue and boost the immune system when used in a
cream – a natural 'anti-ageing' ingredient.

In 1903, Rubinstein advertised it as follows: 'Valaze by
Dr Lykusky, the most celebrated European Skin Specialist, is
the best nourisher of the skin. Valaze will improve the worst
skin in one month ...'[2] A few years later, she dropped the
'Dr Lykusky' character and positioned herself in the role of
'beauty scientist', working steadfastly to create products that
would supposedly help women look 'forever young'.

By the time she died in 1965, Rubinstein had created a
US$60 million beauty empire and, as written by Mark Tungate
in his book *Branded Beauty*, 'it was founded not just on pots of
cream, but also on brilliant, ground-breaking marketing ...
Rubinstein combined the key ingredients of modern beauty
marketing: glossy packaging, celebrity endorsement and
pseudo-science.'[3]

Sound familiar? Nothing much has changed since those early
days in the skincare industry. At the same time as Rubinstein
was building her business, Pond's cold cream went from a
pharmaceutical product to a luxury skincare product via the
power of branding and marketing. Also, around the same time,
Elizabeth Arden created a small line of skincare products with
beautiful packaging and branding in her salon on Fifth Avenue.
Her first major hit was a cream called Venetian Cream Amoretta,
sold with the advertising claim that it had been made from a
famous French formula (which is debatable). Arden intuitively
understood that consumers would believe anything in the
quest for beauty. Her next product was Ardena Skin Tonic,
which cost 5 cents to make (including the label and the bottle)
but sold for 85 cents. That is one heck of a profit margin.

Savvy and shrewd entrepreneurs are not the only people to blame for the rise of Big Skincare. Did doctors, historically, ever sell topical lotions and potions? Yes, of course – and, unfortunately, dermatology and dermatologists have been associated with 'quackery' for over a century.[4] A 'quack' is someone who pretends to have medical knowledge or skill. With many dermatologists and doctors now actively engaging with Big Skincare in the promotion, sale and use of products and treatments with no proven efficacy, we are not helping the reputation of our own speciality (or of medicine in general).

In this section we will be discussing mainly cosmetic skincare – what it is, how it works and the scientific evidence for whether it is 'necessary'. I will also be going into detail about the topical prescription treatments that have a strong scientific evidence base for their intended effect. By the end of this section, you will be armed with the information and facts you need to make a choice about what is best for you when you next need or want to buy a facial cleanser or a moisturiser . . . or (God forbid!) a serum.

The overarching bottom line here is that **most people need very few – if any – skincare products in their daily life. Nothing is essential and a multi-step 'routine' is totally unnecessary**, but if we are going to discuss 'categories' of skincare that you will probably use anyway and are often helpful as adjuvant to treatment, the main three are facial cleansers, moisturisers and sunscreen. We are going to start with those and then move on to talking about all the other diverse products Big Skincare has on offer that you just don't need.

4

Facial Cleansers and Moisturisers

Two questions I get asked on a daily basis are 'What is the best cleanser?' and 'What is the best moisturiser?' And though there is no such thing as 'essential' skincare, facial cleansers and moisturisers are probably the two most commonly purchased and used categories of skincare. However, the number one concern I hear from patients about any skincare product – whether it is a basic moisturiser, cleanser or a prescribed treatment – is 'Will it give me spots?' So, first we need to discuss 'comedogenicity' – the term used to describe the ability of a skincare product or ingredient to cause a break-out or to bring on pimples. To me, this is the most misunderstood concept in skincare, so I want to make sure that we unpack it thoroughly and completely before going any further.

UNDERSTANDING THE CONCEPT OF COMEDOGENICITY

Although the FDA (US Food and Drug Administration) does not have a legal definition for the term 'comedogenic' and there is no actual list of ingredients recognised as such, skincare manufacturers and consumers believe that a product labelled 'non-comedogenic' implies that the final product does not clog facial pores (hair follicles) with skin cells, debris and oil. The concept is that if pores get clogged, this will lead to comedones (pores that have become blocked with bacteria, oil and dead skin cells to form a bump on your skin) and possibly small, inflamed papules (small red bumps) and pustules (bumps filled with pus), known as acne cosmetica (to differentiate it from acne vulgaris, which is an androgen-driven disease of the hair follicle unit – see Chapter 12). It takes four weeks for comedones to form on human facial skin when exposed to pore-clogging products.[1] (Comedogenicity needs to be distinguished from 'acnegenicity' – the idea that a finished skincare product can produce true acne vulgaris. There is no standard test done for acnegenicity, except for use testing. Volunteers use the product as intended for one month and are examined for the presence of papules and pustules.[2])

The concept of comedogenicity entered the world of skincare in 1972 when a paper was published linking adult female acne to the use of cosmetic formulations containing certain ingredients thought to be capable of producing comedones.[3] The uncovering of which chemicals could do this became a mission for Big Skincare, with the development of the poorly conceived 'rabbit ear model' leading to many ingredients being erroneously labelled as 'comedogenic'. Ten years later, a human model for testing comedogenicity was made and gave wildly different results from the rabbit ear model.[4]

Today, only the human model is used and considered reasonably accurate. Typically, the final formulation or ingredient for testing is applied to the upper back of persons capable of forming comedones, daily, for 2–4 weeks. A positive control (a substance guaranteed to cause comedones, like crude coal tar) is applied, and a negative control (a substance guaranteed not to cause comedones, like pure petroleum jelly) is also applied. The comedones are extracted from the upper back and are counted under a microscope. Any increase in comedones following the exposure period deems that product or ingredient to be comedogenic.[5] This is far from a perfect test and it is an exaggeration of real life: the test chemicals or products are used on patients who are known to be prone to acne, the skin on the back has larger hair follicles that are more easily blocked (occluded) than facial skin and the products are placed under occlusion (covered with plasters) for weeks, which is very different from using a skincare product daily on the face!

So, are any ingredients or products truly comedogenic? Yes – the ingredients used as 'positive controls' in human comedogenicity testing. These include crude coal tar, octyl palmitate, isopropyl myristate and acetylated lanolin alcohol, but only when used in high enough concentrations. One study checked the comedogenicity of a variety of skincare products.[6] A face powder, cleanser, moisturiser, sunscreen, day cream, night cream, powder make-up and bronzing powder were all found not to be comedogenic during four weeks of human testing. However, every product tested had at least one ingredient in it that is known to be comedogenic and can be used as a positive control. How is this possible? This occurs because **the concentration of the seemingly comedogenic ingredients is so much lower in the finished products than when the ingredient is tested just on its own.**

There has been a great deal of controversy for decades about how to test if a chemical or substance is comedogenic and whether these findings are even relevant in real life (which, for the most part, they don't appear to be). One thing we know for sure is that the comedogenicity of a substance has nothing to do with how oily or greasy it is; the chemical structure of the compound determines comedogenicity. Some of the most potent 'pore-clogging' substances are not oily at all (like dioxin, an environmental pollutant). The underlying reason why or how a substance is comedogenic is not known.[7]

So, should you be worried about your skincare products or make-up worsening acne or giving you acne cosmetica? Many women use multiple facial products daily and most of these products have virtually the same ingredients in them. This can then theoretically increase the concentration of ingredients known to be comedogenic at high concentrations, perhaps leading to the formation of comedones.

> **The bottom line**: It's the use of multiple products at once that can be a problem, not any one single product.

Importantly, you cannot judge if a product is giving you comedones or aggravating your acne after only a few days of using it. It takes weeks of continued use to see that change. Moreover, it is unlikely that if you are having a comedone problem it is due to just one product; rather it will be due to the use of multiple products being layered at the same time.

SKINTELLIGENT FACT:

A new cosmetic product cannot give you acne vulgaris overnight

'I used that product once and it gave me spots' – I hear this from patients every single day. It has probably happened to you, especially if you have acne-prone skin: you buy a new skincare product, use it and the next day you have one or two or even a crop of new pimples. And you blame it on the new product. But can this really happen?

We already know that it takes four weeks for comedones to form on human facial skin, and pimples start out as comedones. Therefore, it would take at least four weeks for acne to develop from product use. There are, however, certain individuals who will develop tiny papules and pustules within 48 hours of using a skincare product or cosmetic. This is not acne vulgaris or even acne cosmetica - true acne cannot develop in 48 hours. What is happening here is an irritant contact dermatitis that is affecting the hair follicle and surrounding skin. Yes, it may look like acne, but the rapid onset of these monomorphic (all the same size) lesions is due to irritation from the product or products used. This problem is avoided by minimising how many products you use or sticking to products that are very basic, without a lot of 'special' ingredients or 'actives' that may be irritating. As you'll soon see, keep your skincare simple!

The bottom line: Simply choosing a product labelled as 'non-comedogenic' doesn't really mean anything; it is a marketing technique used by Big Skincare to sell products.

CLEANSERS

The goal of cleansing facial skin is to gently remove make-up, skincare products, pollutants from the environment like dust and sweat from the skin surface without causing irritation or excess dryness. In my opinion, cleansing is one of the least important parts of 'skincare' and Big Skincare places far too much emphasis on it. If we didn't wear make-up or sunscreen, then a splash of water would be all that is required to remove any dust or dirt and prepare the skin for the application of any specific treatments. Excessive cleansing, using too much water or rubbing the skin when removing make-up or cleansing are all underestimated in their ability to worsen skin problems like acne vulgaris (see page 163), rosacea (see page 206), dry skin (see page 38) and atopic dermatitis or eczema (see page 218).[8]

All skin cleansers – from foaming cleansers and face washes

to cleansing bars, milks, gels, balms and lotions, and anything else Big Skincare has labelled them as – are based on 'surface-active' substances, also known as 'surfactants', that, when applied to the skin, lower the surface tension at the oil–water interface.[9] Classic soaps are manufactured from fatty acids and alkalis, and hence are alkaline, with a pH of around 9 or 10. They do cause excessive drying of the skin but can be 'superfatted' with the addition of lanolin or glycerol, making them less drying. Beauty or cleansing bars are not actually soap at all but rather detergents with additives like emollients and acids to make them less drying than classic soap. These cleansers with non-soap-based surfactants are referred to as 'syndets' (synthetic detergent-based bars or liquids).[10] Liquid cleansers are basically cleansing bars in liquid form and tend to foam. Cleansing milks are emulsions and are a combination of a liquid cleanser and a cream, containing about 30 per cent oil.

Cleansing should not remove the lipids or oils from the stratum corneum or even excessively from the skin surface, because doing so can lead to problems with irritation, especially if specific treatments or products are applied to the skin surface directly after cleansing. My preference for all my patients is to **use oil-based cleansers because they are very gentle, non-drying and have a higher cleansing ability compared to other cleansers.**[11] Anything that leaves a slight film on your skin that doesn't make your skin feel tight or dry afterwards is good.

Cleansing oils are oils with added surfactants. You apply them to dry skin and, with the addition of a small amount of water, they form into a slight lather or milky consistency, which can then be gently wiped or rinsed away while thoroughly removing make-up and products from the skin surface. Importantly, oil cleansers do not dry out the skin through excessive rinsing or scrubbing. A soft flannel or face wipe can be used to assist in the removal of make-up. And that's it.

SKINTELLIGENT TIP:

Flannels versus face wipes

Are flannels any different from face wipes when it comes to cleansing? Aside from the environmental impact, they aren't. Let's think about this logically.

A face wipe is a soft, disposable cloth made from a combination of polyester, rayon, cotton and cellulose fibres that has been 'impregnated' with a cleanser-type ingredient (you can even buy ones impregnated with only coconut oil!). They are either pre-moistened or come dry and you add water to make a foaming or cream cleanser.

How is this different from using micellar water on a cotton pad? Or any cleanser with a flannel? It's not. There is no physiological reason why cleansing with a flannel is any different from using a face wipe. Just use what you like to use, though wipes are terrible for the environment!

The most important part of cleansing your face is not the cleanser at all: it's the water; 80 per cent of cleansing is achieved by the water alone. Hot water as well as lots of water will remove more of the intercellular lipids than cold water and less water. So, **the best way to cleanse is to apply a few drops of your oil cleanser to your skin, gently rub it in with your fingertips, add some cold water and rinse with a splash or two of cold water**. Colder water is better than hot or lukewarm water because we're trying to protect the skin and treat it gently.

SKINTELLIGENT TIP:

*'Double cleansing' is a concept invented by
Big Skincare*

'Double cleansing' is a fairly new concept that has become popularised as an 'essential' part of skincare routines by seemingly well-meaning but misinformed 'influencers' in the realm of social media and popular skincare media.

The purported benefit is that the first 'cleanse' done with an oil or balm cleanser removes make-up and the second performed with a foaming cleanser removes the 'residue' from the first cleanser and any leftover make-up or products not removed by the first cleanse.

However, as we've seen, less cleansing is generally better because both water and cleansers can negatively impact the skin barrier. There is no need for 'double cleansing' unless it is something you particularly enjoy, but if you are using the correct cleanser for what you need it is unnecessary. The idea of 'double cleansing' is a skincare-industry-invented concept to sell more products and imparts no physiological benefit to skin health and, for some, could even be detrimental.

MOISTURISERS

In 1878 a young American named Harley Procter, along with his chemist cousin James Gamble, developed the first widely marketed cleansing soap – the creamy white soap bar 'Ivory Soap'. In fact, it is the only 'true' soap bar widely available on the market today. They discovered, by accident, that whipping air into the soap solution before moulding it resulted in a floating bar of soap – very convenient for bathing in both bathtubs and the great outdoors. And so began the story of Procter and Gamble, now one of the biggest skincare companies in the world, with global net sales in 2020 of over US$70 billion.[12]

Basic soap is very efficient at removing the lipids in the stratum corneum and increasing the pH of the skin and, as we've seen, both of those changes have a direct effect on the skin's ability to temporarily prevent an increase in transepidermal water loss (TEWL – see page 15). So back in the late 1800s when soap began to be used regularly thanks to Ivory Soap, more people began to develop skin flaking and dryness – which then was a new problem that needed to be fixed. Hence, the concept of the 'moisturiser' came into the world.

The use of bland, non-medicated emollients to treat a variety of skin conditions is as old as dermatology itself. The term 'emollient' comes from the Greek, meaning 'to soften'. The term 'moisturisers' is a creation of Madison Avenue marketeers working for Big Skincare and is generally used to refer to water-based creams. The two terms are now used interchangeably to encompass a huge variety of commercial products.

Despite the long list of obscure ingredients and pseudoscience gibberish you will find with many moisturiser packaging and claims, they all help with dry skin in the same way: by trapping water in the skin and temporarily softening and smoothing the stratum corneum. They do not impart anything significant that is 'moisturising' to the skin itself – they just stop water loss. Expensive moisturisers are not better for skin; the most expensive parts of any cosmetic product are the packaging and the fragrance, neither of which affect the actual ability of the product to moisturise. If greasiness weren't a problem, everyone would just use basic ointments like petroleum jelly since it is the best at trapping water in the skin. In fact, the very first moisturiser was pure petroleum jelly, known worldwide by its brand name Vaseline.

Oily occlusive products containing petrolatum, paraffin, mineral oil and dimethicone create a film (acting as a seal) across the skin surface to decrease evaporation of water from the skin, therefore increasing the water content of the skin. Products containing humectants that draw water in, such as glycerine, sorbitol, propylene glycol and urea, attract water to the top layers of the skin from either the atmosphere or deeper layers of the skin.

You will probably be familiar with the different types of moisturisers on the market, but for completeness we will just run through them:

- A *cream* is equal parts water and oil.
- A *lotion*, in dermatology, is a watery liquid used as a scalp application, but in lay terminology it is usually a thinner, runnier version of a cream.
- A *gel* is usually a clear jelly-like substance made of a liquid with a three-dimensional cross-linked polymer dissolved in it.
- A *serum* is a term invented by the skincare industry to describe a low-viscosity (thin) oil and water combination (not a moisturiser at all).

The majority of popular commercial moisturisers have water as the first ingredient. But the water isn't there to hydrate the skin – it's part of the vehicle and evaporates when applied, possibly drying the skin further. When you apply a water-based moisturiser to your skin, you are repeatedly wetting and drying the skin surface, which potentially over time further damages already dry skin.

If you are caught in a cycle of thinking your skin constantly feels dry if you don't use a water-based moisturiser, this is almost certainly what is happening. That is one of the (many) reasons I suggest that my patients use an ointment (anything that has a lip balm texture and without water or 'aqua' listed as an ingredient) instead of a water-based cream, but especially if they are undergoing treatment with retinoids for acne or the treatment of fine lines, or any other initially irritating prescription treatment, like acids or benzoyl peroxide. I recognise that these types of moisturisers are heavier, stickier and shiny, so you may opt to only use them at night after you use your prescription treatment.

SKINTELLIGENT TIP:

Silicones do not prevent the absorption of actives

Silicones are ubiquitous in skincare products, with dimethicone and cyclopentasiloxane the two most used. You may have recently heard that silicones reduce the amount of active ingredients that the skin can absorb – some cosmetic manufacturers even claim that their products are superior because they don't have any silicone in them! This is incorrect.

Silicones in skincare are neither good nor bad: they do a job in your skincare product, and they most likely need to be there. The compounded creams I prescribe usually have some sort of silicone in the vehicle. Dimethicone is a silicone-based polymer that is in all 'oil-free' moisturisers because it works well as an occlusive and has good emollient characteristics, filling in skin surface imperfections to create a smooth appearance. It is the second most used ingredient in moisturisers after petrolatum because it doesn't give as greasy a feel to the skin.

So don't worry about silicone in your skincare product – it does not impair the active ingredients penetrating the skin and it doesn't clog your pores.

Emollients are not technically medicines so they do not contain any pharmacologically active substances. That being said, some emollients do more than just soften and moisten. The one that stands out is good old Vaseline.

Learn to love Vaseline

Sir Robert Chesebrough was a London-born, New York-bred chemist. When petroleum was discovered in Pennsylvania, he created petroleum jelly ('petrolatum' or 'pure petrolatum'), patented it and called it 'Vaseline'. The word 'Vaseline' is an amalgamation of the German word for water and the ancient Greek word for oil.

Petroleum jelly is an occlusive that traps water in the skin, forms a layer over damaged skin, stopping dirt from getting into a wound (infected open wounds were one of the leading causes of death back in the day) and keeps skin hydrated by reducing transepidermal water loss.

Though a massive fan of petroleum jelly, arguably the most well-known and influential dermatologist of all time, Dr Albert Kligman, admitted in the last paper he wrote before he died that the biggest issue with patients using petroleum jelly is its 'greasiness and disagreeable feel'.[13] As emollients like ointments are superior to water-based lotions or creams, after experimenting with a variety of ointments he concluded that Aquaphor Soothing Skin Balm, made by Eucerin and available commercially throughout the world, comes second only to petrolatum for repairing defective skin barriers in patients with chronic skin disease. He stressed that patients need to be taught to rub it in properly, so that the greasy feeling all but disappears.

So how does petroleum jelly help improve a variety of the chronic inflammatory conditions we treat in dermatology, like atopic eczema?

Petroleum jelly has anti-inflammatory properties

In the 1970s it was found that petroleum jelly functioned as an anti-inflammatory agent when applied to skin. A groundbreaking study in 1976 was the first time petroleum jelly was shown to reduce inflammation in real-life skin disease, specifically in chronic plaque psoriasis (where skin cells pile up on the surface of the skin – see page 22). The 'Koebner phenomenon' is the development of psoriasis plaques in traumatised but otherwise unaffected skin of patients with active psoriasis. In the study, uninvolved skin was pretreated with petroleum jelly for three weeks before attempting to provoke the Koebner phenomenon with a 1-cm-long deep scratch. No new psoriasis plaques formed, presumably due to the inhibitory effect of pretreating with petroleum jelly.[14]

Dr Kligman investigated the ability of emollients to inhibit UV-induced tumour formation in hairless mice. He applied a specific emollient to each hairless mouse right before irradiating them 3 times a week for 20 weeks with broad-spectrum UVB. He found, remarkably, that petroleum jelly gave almost complete protection again the formation of tumours. By contrast, lanolin was only 50 per cent effective and mineral oil greatly enhanced tumour formation, possibly because it is not as occlusive as petroleum jelly. Cold cream had no protective effect.[15]

Petroleum jelly has been found to be beneficial in a number of clinical settings including after chemical and laser peels, after dermabrasion, in promoting wound healing and, of course, in soothing chronic, inflammatory skin disease.

Petroleum jelly enhances the repair of a damaged skin barrier

In one study, six different moisturisers were examined for their ability to repair the stratum corneum after it was damaged by a 24-hour patch test of 0.5 per cent sodium lauryl sulphate (SLS).[16]

(Note: the authors state quite clearly even in the abstract of the paper that *'no commercial interests were involved in the study'* – that's not something you see stated so categorically in skincare publications!) SLS is a chemical used as a detergent in lots of skincare products (mainly cleansers) that makes the barrier extremely permeable (allowing liquids to pass through it), increasing TEWL by 20 times. All six moisturisers tested accelerated barrier repair after five days of three-times-a-day application of a 'thin layer', with petrolatum being the best performer. A key finding of the study was that the greasier the moisturiser, the more effective it was at repairing the skin barrier.

This shows that petroleum jelly accelerates rather than delays barrier recovery after it has been disrupted; it doesn't just sit on top of the skin like a layer of plastic – it also integrates into the intercellular pathways at all levels of the stratum corneum and allows for normal barrier recovery despite its occlusive properties.

Petroleum jelly is safe

Petroleum jelly is actually a very complex mixture of hundreds of saturated hydrocarbons and it is produced by the fractional distillation of petroleum. It is refined exhaustively to remove colour, aromatic hydrocarbons and impurities. The brand-name Vaseline you buy in the shops (made by Unilever) is very safe.

SKINTELLIGENT FACT:

Petroleum jelly does not clog pores

In 1996, Dr Kligman performed a study to see whether petroleum jelly clogged pores. He had 20 patients with moderate acne (defined as having at least 10

---

papules/pustules and 15 comedones on their faces at the time the trial started) use either Vaseline (100 per cent petrolatum) or a 30 per cent petrolatum cream in a pea-sized amount twice daily to their entire face and no other products, aside from a mild soap to cleanse, for 8 weeks.

He found that both groups had a significant reduction in papules/pustules from baseline. Comedone numbers did not decrease but they *did not increase* either. Even more importantly, not a single subject had worsening acne.

As Kligman wrote: '[Acne] patients are urged to seek oil-free cosmetics. This advice has *not* been supported by scientific studies. Comedogenicity has nothing whatever to do with oiliness; the latter is a physical attribute and not a chemical entity.'

Petroleum jelly is well-known for being non-comedogenic and there is zero evidence to suggest that mineral oil or petroleum jelly clogs pores or contributes to acne. This was reiterated at the American Academy of Dermatology symposium on comedogenicity in 1989.[17]

Moisturising 'normal' skin

Theoretically and according to some study findings, a moisturiser can delay barrier recovery if applied regularly to normal skin. Remember that the effect described above was when Vaseline was applied to irritated or damaged skin. This brings up a very important question: can the regular use of a moisturiser on entirely normal skin cause problems? A group of dermatologists investigated this exact issue.[18] They had healthy volunteers apply a petroleum jelly-based moisturiser three times a day to one forearm for four weeks (the other forearm was not treated and was used as the control). After the four weeks, both forearms were challenged with SLS.

They found that TEWL was significantly higher post-challenge on the arm treated with moisturiser than on the control arm. These results suggest that the long-term use of moisturisers on normal skin may increase susceptibility to irritants and could theoretically interfere with the lipid matrix of the stratum corneum (see page 19), resulting in a change in the barrier function of the skin. When the moisturiser is stopped, the barrier function is potentially compromised, making it more susceptible to irritation. **This throws into doubt the general idea that the daily use of moisturisers on normal skin increases hydration levels by reducing TEWL, therefore 'improving' the overall 'health' of normal skin.**

Data on the effect of moisturisers on TEWL are also contradictory. In one study, a moisturiser that contained urea decreased TEWL after three weeks of use on both dry and normal skin.[19] Another study found that TEWL remained constant after seven days of treatment.[20] In normal skin, the use of any moisturiser should not affect TEWL at all because normal skin by definition has normal barrier function.

> **The bottom line**: If you have totally normal skin, you may be better off not moisturising at all. Like the old adage states, 'if it ain't broke, don't fix it'.

Moisturising for skin diseases

Traditional moisturiser ingredients like lanolin, glycerol and petrolatum generally increase hydration in the skin by creating a barrier to TEWL by both sitting on top of the skin and filling up the spaces between the corneocytes in the stratum corneum. However, they do not reach the viable epidermis. (See pages 13–32 for a refresher on the structure of the skin.)

In certain skin diseases, like atopic dermatitis or eczema, we know that the quantity of lipids in the stratum corneum is reduced, which is one reason for the visible signs of dryness in these conditions. To fix this problem, moisturisers have been created that have fats in them in the same or similar mixture as that found in the skin – these are referred to as 'physiological lipid-based moisturisers'. The most well-known moisturiser that does this is ceramide-based.

There are many studies demonstrating the safety and efficacy of barrier repair products, either as a single therapy or used alongside other topicals, like steroids, in the treatment of eczema. These 'special' moisturisers are usually only available on prescription and are generally very expensive. However, are they superior to ordinary over-the-counter moisturisers? That's the £50 million question! Two studies compared prescription barrier repair moisturisers to regular standard emollients in patients with eczema, and neither found a difference between the two types of moisturisers in their ability to improve the eczema.[21]

> **The bottom line**: If you have a skin problem, using specifically marketed barrier repair products isn't going to make a difference.

Are all brands of moisturiser the same?

If you look at the breakdown below you will see that the similarities have to do with what a moisturiser *does*, and the differences have to do with how it *feels* or *looks*.

Similarities	Differences
Composition: combination of occlusives, emollients and humectants	Consistency (feel): greasy, light, sticky, etc. (subjective)
Ingredients: glycerin, urea, paraffins, water, preservatives, emulsifiers	Marketing claims: oil-free, anti-ageing, anti-redness, all-natural

Similarities	Differences
Soften/smooth skin temporarily by increasing or preserving water in the stratum corneum	Packaging
	Price point
	Use of fragrances

Most people buy a moisturiser for what it does – moisturise. The level of moisturisation is a direct consequence of the consistency of the product. **A greasier moisturiser improves skin hydration more than a less greasy lotion or cream. And a non-water-based ointment will have fewer or no preservatives in it, making it less likely to irritate skin**, especially when the skin is inflamed or irritated due to a skin disease or product use.

So, which brand of moisturiser should you use? Whichever you like and can afford because, in the end, they all do the same thing – they all moisturise to one degree or another ('hydrate' by reducing TEWL). With something more watery and less greasy you will find you need to reapply it more often to get the same level of constant hydration you would achieve by using a greasier ointment and applying it just once daily.

I recommend all my patients use ointment-based moisturisers like Vaseline because they are the best at trapping water in the skin and the least likely to cause irritation. But I also appreciate that a lot of people don't like the greasy feel, so I recommend using the greasier ointments at night and, if necessary, a lighter-weight water-based cream during the day. Ointments are so hydrating, though, that my patients often find they don't need a moisturiser during the day at all! **The best way to apply an ointment is to first put a thin layer on your hands, rub your hands together to make it soft and just pat it on your face.**

The case of Chanel in Sweden

Big Skincare will make you believe that the more you spend on a moisturiser, the better it will be for your skin. Though we all recognise that, with certain things, price and quality are linked (though finding an example of this today can be challenging), it is certainly not the case with cosmetic skincare. Branding and packaging can make you think a more expensive product is more effective, but is it?

A group of dermatologists in Sweden actually went so far as to do a clinical trial to understand if the branding and packaging of a facial moisturiser would have any effect on product use or how well it was perceived to 'work'.[22] The subjects were asked to use a facial moisturiser twice a day for six weeks, while sticking to their normal make-up and cleanser routine. The subjects were randomly allocated to three groups to each receive a different cream: group A got a brand-new jar of Chanel Precision Ultra Correction Restructuring Anti-Wrinkle Firming Cream SPF 10 (retail price £105 for 50ml). Group B was given the same Chanel jar and packaging, but the Chanel cream itself was replaced by a generic, inexpensive moisturiser (ACO Facial Cream, retail price £15.75 for 50ml) matched for colour to the original Chanel cream. The third group, group C, was given the real Chanel cream in a plain white jar.

At the end of the six weeks, groups A and B – the ones using the cream in the Chanel packaging – had used significantly more cream than group C. Group B rated the absorption of their cream (the cheap cream) as significantly better than the other two groups and they were more likely to find that their cream was a 'luxury' cream. Over 50 per cent of all the subjects did not think the creams – any of them – improved the appearance of their wrinkles. The trained observer did not find any significant differences in the clinical signs of ageing between any of the groups after six weeks.

The bottom line: Expensive moisturisers are definitely not better at 'moisturising' or improving the appearance of wrinkles than cheap ones.

SKINTELLIGENT TIP:

Coconut oil is a good moisturiser

There are three studies that have shown that coconut oil reduces TEWL in both newborns and adults, without irritation, to a similar or slightly greater extent when compared to pure mineral oil.[23] In addition, coconut oil is primarily made of lauric acid, which is believed to have both anti-inflammatory and anti-microbial properties. So, if you like coconut oil, go ahead and use it as a moisturiser for your face and body, but make sure it is a high-quality virgin coconut oil; coconut oil derivatives (cocamidopropyl betaine, cocamide diethanolamine), as commonly found in cosmetic skincare products, are known to cause allergic contact dermatitis in some people and are not the same thing as pure virgin coconut oil.

PRIVATE-LABEL PRODUCTS

There's a common myth in the skincare industry – and it's perhaps even more pervasive among those on the outside of it, looking in – that every brand has its own army of formulators and scientists toiling away in some high-tech lab creating its products. And while that may be true for a handful of them, the reality is that many of those products are researched, created and packaged by private-label companies.

Private-label companies are B2B (business-to-business) manufacturers that create formulas and packaging that can be marketed by skincare brands without anyone knowing they didn't do it themselves. Consumers might be surprised to learn that some of their favourite lotions and potions come from the same place and potentially have the same formula as other private-label-produced products on the market.

It is, of course, impossible to know how many of the skincare products available on the market today are manufactured by private-label companies, but it is certainly a good number of them. This presents a problem for the consumer: what are you paying for when you buy an expensive skincare product?

When you spend a lot of money on a product from an expensive, luxury skincare brand that has used a private-label manufacturer, it is like you have gone to the Ritz-Carlton for dinner, ordered pommes frites (French fries or chips to you and me) and the chef went out to McDonald's, bought some large fries for £1.99, brought it to his kitchen at the Ritz, arranged them on a fancy plate with a drizzle of truffle oil and some green leaves on the side and charged you £14.99 for them. Those fries might look all fancy and high-end, but really you have just paid a lot of money for standard McDonald's French fries; they taste good and do the job, but they are not the quality, hand-crafted, 'premium' deep-fried potatoes you think you are paying for.

Basically, you have been tricked: the fancy surroundings, the presentation and the high price make you believe that what you are getting is special and potentially 'super effective'. And you will hold on to this manufactured belief for a good few weeks until you forget all about the lovely experience and you start to realise that the chips weren't really anything special, you start to ask yourself 'why did I spend so much on them?' and the buyer's remorse and regret invariably follow.

Most private-label companies divide their stock into 'tiers' – like some designer fashion labels do. There's 'ready-to-wear', in which brands pick an existing product from the available stock line. This is the cheapest option, because these products already have names given to them by the private-label company along with its packaging, but they also add on the new brand's logo and info.

The next tier also offers product and packaging drawn from the stock options, but the company adds custom labels with the brand's colour scheme, chosen product name and logo, making it look like the brand's own proprietary product.

Then there's the more premium option – or couture, if we stick with fashion terms – which is a custom formulation, that could simply be a reformulation of an existing product, a reverse-engineered formula (or, to put it more bluntly, a knock-off) or a fully bespoke formulation built from the ground up.

One of the big private-label manufacturers uses this as their website strapline: 'we'll take care of the cosmetics, so you can focus on growth'.

Because of the existence of private-label companies, virtually anyone with a spare £15–20K and a marketing 'vision' can start a skincare line. On the other hand, manufacturing a product 'from scratch' can take months and literally tens of thousands of pounds. And since most skincare products are virtually identical anyway, why would anyone choose not to use a private-label manufacturer, with their ready-made cleansers and moisturisers, just waiting for a fancy new bottle, label, claim and hefty price tag to be attached to them?

You can see why skincare start-ups opt for private label over starting from scratch. And skincare is, of course, extremely lucrative – all the money not used to create a skincare product from scratch goes into branding and PR, and, thanks to social media, small start-up companies are able to flog copycat or basic products at a high price point and make a massive return – as long as they have their marketing and branding spot-on.

How much does it cost to make one bottle of cleanser via private label? And then how much is it sold for? You are paying a thousand times the cost of the actual manufacturing for a skincare product that is the equivalent of Tesco's own-brand baked beans. And we thought Starbucks was a rip-off.

But you can't compare private labelling to own-brand private labelling of food – in the food industry, own-brand is done to offer a cheaper but hopefully almost equivalent product in keeping with the brand of the supermarket. But universally these own-brand private-label products will be cheaper than the 'big name' brands. That is not the case in skincare – in fact, it is often the reverse. The small, new, 'niche' skincare brands that have sprung up over the past few years are generally more expensive than the big brands while offering a standard, or almost identical, product . . . just in newer, on-trend packaging.

That rounds up the Skintelligent approach to facial cleansers and moisturisers. Let's now look at the science and evidence base around the use of sunscreen.

5

Sunscreen

S kin cancer is the most commonly diagnosed cancer in Europe and the United States. Excess sun exposure is the most significant risk factor for developing skin cancer, as well as accounting for 90 per cent of age-associated cosmetic skin problems. In addition, Big Skincare is a multi-billion-dollar empire focused on providing treatments for UV-light-induced signs of ageing skin, like dark spots, fine lines and coarse skin texture. For both these reasons, sunscreen use is becoming more and more widespread, with sunscreens now ubiquitous in daily-use moisturisers, make-up and even lip gloss. It has been estimated that the incidence of both short- and long-term hazards of UV radiation can be reduced by nearly 80 per cent over a person's lifetime if sunscreens are applied to the skin properly from the age of 6 months until 18 years of age.[1]

Solar radiation comes from the sun (stating the obvious, I know) and 95 per cent of this is UVA (320–400nm), which is not filtered by the ozone and damages the skin via the formation of free radicals, which is why it is often referred to as the 'ageing' rays. The other 5 per cent is UVB (290–320nm), the 'burning' rays, and.it damages the skin through damaging the DNA of skin cells.[2]

There are two types of sunscreens:

1. Physical (mineral) sunscreens (zinc oxide, titanium dioxide) work by scattering and reflecting UV light. They are inert, sit on your skin, do not break down over time

or in the sun and generally do not cause allergic reactions.

2. Chemical sunscreens work by absorbing UV light through a photochemical reaction. They degrade with sun exposure and therefore require reapplication every 2–3 hours. They also carry a 0.1–2 per cent risk of giving you an allergic reaction.[3]

All sunscreens have an 'SPF' factor. SPF stands for 'sun protection factor' and is the time in minutes you can expose yourself to the sun without getting a burn, and it only relates to the effects of UVB. SPF15 blocks 93 per cent of UVB rays, SPF30 blocks 97 per cent of UVB rays and SPF50 blocks 98 per cent of UVB rays. You also need to check the UVA star rating to make sure you are using a product that covers both types of UV light.

HOW TO CORRECTLY USE SUNSCREEN

There are two aspects to applying sunscreen properly: volume and frequency.

You need to apply $2mg/cm^2$ of skin to achieve the labelled SPF rating. For an average face/neck/ears, that is 2.5ml or ½ a teaspoon. For an average adult body, that is 6 full teaspoons, which is 36g (including the face) – the equivalent of a shot glass. And if using a chemical sunscreen or if you are sweating or swimming, this needs to be reapplied every 2–3 hours. If you are going on a sunny holiday, you are going to need to reapply your sunscreen three times per day, which is 108ml of sunscreen per day. For seven days you will need to pack at least 756ml of sunscreen ... and even more if you have a family!

Unfortunately, most people only use half the amount required to get adequate coverage; that means instead of an SPF30 level of protection you are actually getting an SPF15.

Generally, sunscreen should be good for up to three years after purchase, even after it has been opened. But if you are using enough volume often enough, it should not last you that long.

SKINTELLIGENT TIP:

An oil-based cleanser is best at removing sunscreen

A brilliant study that investigated whether a foaming or oil cleanser is better at removing both normal and waterproof sunscreen was recently published.[4] The foaming cleanser and the oil cleanser were equally good at removing over 85 per cent of the non-waterproof sunscreen. But when it came to removing the waterproof sunscreen, the oil cleanser removed over 94 per cent of it while the foaming cleanser could only get just over 60 per cent of it off! Almost half of the participants reported having dry skin after washing with the foaming cleanser, while only one participant reported that after oil cleansing.

WHAT IS THE BEST SUNSCREEN?

The one you are going to use! Your choice of sunscreen comes down to personal preference and what is affordable to you. Having said that, I recommend getting a non-expensive mineral-based sunscreen, though I would also strongly advise using physical methods of protecting your skin, such as wearing a wide-brimmed hat and big sunglasses, and not lying out in the sun for hours. All these things will go a long way to protecting you not only from skin cancer, but also from the ageing effects of UV light exposure.

Some key points about mineral sunscreens that I often get asked about include:

- Mineral sunscreens do not need to be 'tinted' to work – the colour of the particles does not alter the ability of the minerals to reflect light.
- Mineral sunscreens go on white because the particle size of the mineral is big enough to see, but as it dries it does not look as white. That doesn't mean it's no longer there or has evaporated.
- Though mineral sunscreens are generally considered 'better' than chemical sunscreens, in practice because the mineral ones are harder to spread and less cosmetically acceptable, they tend to provide about 50 per cent less protection than the equivalent chemical sunscreen.

The British Association of Dermatologists recommends a sunscreen with an SPF of at least 30 and a UVA star rating of 4 or 5 – this would classify the sunscreen as 'broad spectrum'.[5]

SKINTELLIGENT TIP:

How to optimise vitamin D production

Vitamin D is essential for bone health and we get it via our diet and sunlight exposure. Prolonged exposure to strong sunlight (leading to burning or tanning) does *not* lead to excess production of vitamin D, because your body has a mechanism for destroying excess vitamin D if it is produced. For optimal vitamin D production, exposure of the arms and legs (with an SPF on the face) for about 5-30 minutes between 10am and 3pm twice a week is sufficient for vitamin D synthesis. This 5-30-minute window is wide because the exact time depends on how dark the skin is naturally (longer periods of exposure are needed for those with darker skin), time of day, season, latitude and the person's age. The time needed to make sufficient vitamin D is typically short and less than the amount of time needed for skin to redden and burn.

Important fact: you can't increase your vitamin D by using sunbeds because sunbeds emit high levels of UVA, and vitamin D is produced in the skin in response to UVB - so sunbeds don't help you make more vitamin D, but they do increase your risk of skin cancer.

The 'global issue' of vitamin D deficiency is a very controversial one. The UK Scientific Advisory Committee on Nutrition recommends a nutrient intake of 400iu per day for most people over four years old, all year round - but that includes intake from all dietary sources (supplements, natural foods like oily fish and fortified foods like fat spreads).[6]

THE MOST COMMON QUESTIONS I GET ASKED ABOUT SUNSCREEN

Do office workers need to reapply sunscreen every 2–3 hours?

A study was recently done to answer this exact question. They had 20 healthy volunteers apply 1g of sunscreen (so that's a dose of 2mg/cm² – two fingertip units!) mixed with 2 per cent invisible blue fluorescent agent onto their faces in the morning.

Photographs were taken with a UV mode at 8am and then every two hours thereafter until 4pm and outdoor activity was limited to less than one hour. Six areas of the face were analysed using digital image analysis software.

The amount of sunscreen reduction was 16.3 per cent at two hours and that was the greatest reduction seen. In total, the sunscreen reduction was 28.2 per cent at the end of the eight-hour day.

The bottom line: If you work indoors and apply the correct volume of sunscreen in the morning, you are still protected by the end of the day and reapplication is unnecessary.[7] This is probably because, while indoors, the sunscreen does not break down like it would if you were outside all day.

If you layer sunscreens, can you add together the SPFs?

Though this might seem logical, it doesn't actually happen. If you do layer products containing SPF – and assuming you are using the correct volume to achieve the stated SPF on the product – the SPF you achieve will be that of the product with the highest SPF.

Let me break it down:

You first apply your SPF50 sunscreen, which blocks 98 per cent of UVB rays. Then you apply a foundation with SPF15 in it, which blocks 93 per cent of UVB, and then you brush on an SPF30 powder, which blocks 97 per cent of UVB.

Your final SPF will be 50 – blocking 98 per cent of UVB rays. This is the most protection you will get and that won't increase no matter how many products you put on. Even SPF100 can't block 100 per cent of UVB rays.

However, layering sunscreen is not a bad idea because it does increase your chances of putting enough on to cover your whole face just in case you missed a spot somewhere. Just remember that it won't increase your overall protection. Your best bet is to aim to use the right volume (2.5ml) to cover your entire face to try to achieve the stated SPF.

Are sunscreens regulated?

All sunscreens with the same SPF and UVA star rating should technically offer the same level of protection, if applied correctly, so it should not matter if the sunscreen costs £2 or £200, or if it is a cream, gel or lotion. That's because sunscreens are strictly regulated globally for efficacy and safety, but to what extent and how they are labelled depends on where in the world you live.

In the EU, sunscreen products are classified as cosmetics and defined as: 'any preparation intended to be placed in contact with the human skin with a view exclusively or mainly to protecting it from UV radiation by absorbing, scattering or reflecting radiation'.[8] Sunscreen products must protect against both UVA and UVB rays and there are standard approved testing protocols that the European Commission requires of manufacturers to demonstrate any sunscreen product sold in the EU provides the stated protection levels.

In the United States, sunscreens are classified as over-the-counter drugs, so they are regulated and require pre-market registration via the FDA (just like prescription medicines). And the FDA doesn't mess around, so if you buy a sunscreen in the United States, you can be confident that it will provide the level of protection it says on the bottle.

Are chemical sunscreens safe for daily, lifelong use?

In 2019, the first exploratory maximal usage trial (MUsT) evaluating the absorption through the skin and into the body of the active chemical ingredients in four commercially available sunscreen products was published.[9] A MUsT study assesses the systemic (whole-body) absorption of a topical drug or product when it is used according to the maximum limit of the product's directions for use.

In the study, all six of the chemicals tested showed absorption into the body greater than 0.5ng/mL. The active ingredients that were tested were avobenzone, oxybenzone, octocrylene, homosalate, octisalate and octinoxate.

So, what does this mean for you? Well, nothing – at the moment. We don't know anything about the clinical significance of this finding, such as whether it matters that sunscreen is absorbed into the body or whether it has any impact on health. This is not an excuse not to wear sunscreen. If you are concerned, you could switch to using a physical (mineral) sunscreen made of zinc oxide or titanium dioxide. Otherwise, please keep using sunscreen as you have been as there is currently no evidence to suggest that using chemical sunscreen is dangerous.

Is SPF100 better than SPF50?

SPF100 is indeed better at protecting from sunburn than SPF50. This was shown in a high-quality clinical trial with 199 participants, using a split-face design so each person used either SPF50 or 100 on each side of their face.[10] Both sunscreens were standard 'big-brand' broad-spectrum inexpensive chemical sunscreens that are easily available in most countries.

The participants applied the sunscreens and then spent an average of six hours out skiing in Vail, Colorado. The next day they were examined to see which side of their face got more sunburnt. The investigators found that over 40 per cent of participants were sunburnt on the SPF50 side compared to 13 per cent on the SPF100 side.

The participants weren't even very good at putting on the sunscreen; despite getting clear instructions, they applied only half the amount of sunscreen required to reach the stated SPF and more than 70 per cent of the participants reported one or fewer reapplications over a six-hour period.

My question is – if they had applied the correct volume of sunscreen, would the SPF50 group still have got sunburnt? And would the SPF100 group not have got sunburnt at all? Considering the fact that most people use nowhere near enough sunscreen volume to achieve the stated SPF, should we all opt for SPF100? Based on this study, I would say yes.

Does blue light damage skin?

If you have ever used a phone or a computer, you may have wondered what the effect of blue light – the predominant light shining from our favourite screens – could be doing to your skin. Capitalising on this, some sunscreen manufacturers have even started claiming that their sunscreen protects against blue light damage. Is this legit? Does blue light damage skin and, if it does, do you need a special sunscreen 24/7 to protect yourself from it?

Blue light refers to visible light with a wavelength of 390–460nm (UVA – the 'ageing' part of sunlight – is 320–400nm). These wavelength ranges are very close to each other, so can blue light damage skin and lead to photoageing? It is important to remember that sunlight in the same spectrum is up to 1,000 times more intense than the blue light emitted from your screens.[11]

Researchers carried out a study looking at the clinical and histological (examined under a microscope) effects of blue light on normal skin.[12] They had eight volunteers have part of their bum skin treated with blue light every day for five days. Biopsies were taken of the treated area. They did not find that the blue light caused DNA damage or any histological signs of photoageing compared to untreated skin.

This study looked at short-term effects of blue light in a small group of subjects. To my knowledge, the long-term effects have not been studied on human facial skin. What I would say is the amount of irradiation coming from our screens is so low that even over time it is probably not going to substantially affect the appearance of the skin.

Do you need to wear sunscreen indoors?

There has been some research that 'suggests' that visible light can cause free radical damage the way that UVA light does and therefore could potentially contribute to skin ageing. Visible light (including blue light) with a wavelength above 400nm probably *does* contribute to skin ageing and carcinogenesis (the formation of cancer) but mostly during *direct* sunlight exposure.

There is no need to wear sunscreen indoors because chemical sunscreen does not block the visible wavelength of light – even if applied at the recommended 2mg/cm^2 required dosage. Mineral sunscreen *does* block visible light, though I am not saying you need to wear sunscreen indoors![13] It is also crucial to recognise that indoor light intensities are much weaker than that of direct sun exposure.

Having looked at how using sunscreen, alongside things like wide-brimmed hats, big sunglasses and not lying out in the sun for hours at a time, will help to protect you from skin cancer and the ageing effects of UV light exposure, let's now look at those products touted by Big Skincare that you definitely don't need in your 'skincare routine'!

6

Skincare Products You Don't Need

There are a number of categories of skincare products and devices that no one needs – ever. In this chapter, I will go through these one by one and explain why you absolutely do not need any of these types of products (though if you do not have skin issues and enjoy using them and they don't cause you any problems, then go for it!).

TONER

Toners, also known as 'astringents', have been a part of a 'three-step' skincare routine for decades. They are meant to be applied on a cotton pad or ball after cleansing to supposedly remove any cleanser residue or oil left behind. They often produce a tight feeling after cleansing that some people like. Toners made for oily skin have alcohol in them to further aid this temporary 'tight' feeling and some even contain menthol to impart a tingling sensation. Regardless of the type you use or even why you feel you use it, toners are completely unnecessary and are probably harmful by further stripping the skin of oil and disrupting the stratum corneum. Just use a decent oil-based cleanser (see page 68) and ditch the toner.[1]

EYE CREAM

I spent a good few hours one day looking at a dozen face creams and the same brands' eye cream offerings. In all the products I looked at, the ingredients on the two products were virtually identical. The main difference was the inclusion of a sunscreen in the face cream and the 'richness' of the product. Face creams tend to have more urea, paraffin and glycerine in them, making them 'greasier' for the most part, while eye creams tend to have more silica, mica or dimethicone, presumably to help them give the illusion of smoothing the skin around the eyes temporarily and imparting a 'lighter' texture.

The idea that eye creams are formulated to be less irritating was not evident from looking at the ingredients; all the products I looked at had the same type of preservatives and fragrances as the corresponding face cream.

This is probably the number one reason why 'eye creams' are totally unnecessary: because they are virtually identical in composition to regular standard face moisturisers. Literally the only difference between face cream and eye cream is the size of the pot and the corresponding price tag; the face cream is usually always better value!

So please **don't waste your money buying a separate eye cream – just dab your face cream around your eyes**. Eye cream is a marketing invention to sell you more products, but this time in cute little (expensive) jars and tubes.

EXFOLIANTS AND SCRUBS

You never need to exfoliate your facial skin. Big Skincare will have you believe that you need to 'help' your stratum corneum shed with the use of specific products. This is just not true; normal skin cells shed daily and are continually being replaced (see page 15). The growth or turnover of the epidermis does not stop after a certain thickness of cells is reached at the stratum corneum. In normal, healthy skin the stratum corneum remains a uniform thickness, not because new cells are not being added but because the keratinised cells at the top of the skin are being lost at a rate equal to their formation. This is the 'natural exfoliation' of the skin and why you don't need to exfoliate skin yourself with a scrub, peel or microdermabrasion gadget. Your skin is self-exfoliating.

There is a family of genetic diseases called ichthyosis in which the keratinocytes (skin cells) are produced at a normal rate and mature normally to form the stratum corneum, but they do not separate normally and do not shed at the surface of the skin. This results in a build-up of scale. Ichthyosis vulgaris is the most common form and affects 1 in 250 people (but usually not the entire skin surface, just parts of it) and most often goes undiagnosed because people think they just have dry skin and don't seek medical attention. The condition is due to a gene defect leading to defective production of filaggrin, which is a protein found in corneocytes that helps maintain the structure and function of the stratum corneum (see page 14). These people still don't need to mechanically exfoliate with scrubs; using a moisturiser with an acid in it like glycolic acid works very well and is less irritating to the skin.

MECHANICAL CLEANSING DEVICES

Mechanical cleansing devices have been adapted from the design of the electric toothbrush and add a level of sophistication to cleansing you can't get from using just your hands or a washcloth or even a standard bristle brush. In theory, the mechanical cleansing devices are meant to provide a more 'thorough' cleanse than conventional methods. But do they? This is highly device- and user-dependent, but in general I would say no. Indeed, they are almost certainly too harsh for daily use and can cause irritation and dryness by disrupting the skin barrier more than the water and cleanser do already. Plus, using one of these devices almost certainly prolongs the cleansing ritual, which, as we've seen, is not only unnecessary but potentially disruptive for skin health (see page 68).

'NATURAL' SKINCARE

The concept of the superiority of 'natural' remedies has always struck me as a bit odd because that means that there must be 'artificial' remedies as well. What is an 'artificial' remedy? Is that something that is manufactured as opposed to growing on the earth? Is a topical retinoid not 'natural' because this vitamin A derivative is made in a lab? Is a 'natural' remedy not made in a lab?

Just because a skincare product claims to be 'natural' means absolutely nothing. That product still had to be made in a lab with preservatives and chemicals – both organic and potentially inorganic – to make it a viable and stable product that sits on the shelf of a store.

> **The bottom line**: Don't buy into the marketing hype – organic or natural or artificial or plant-based, these are just words used by marketing people to make you believe their skincare product is different from and better than the rest.

KOREAN SKINCARE

Korean skincare is based on the concept of a ten-step skincare routine:

1. make-up remover/oil cleanser
2. water-based cleanser
3. exfoliator
4. toner

5. essence
6. treatments
7. sheet masks
8. eye cream
9. moisturiser
10. sun protection

Hmmmm ... I could write a whole chapter about each step explaining exactly why it is unnecessary for skin health, and about how this is a very good example of cultural appropriation.

If you have read this far, you know what I think about skincare routines: simple is always best. Focus on targeted prescription products for your skincare complaint. Everything else is unnecessary. The idea of a ten-step skincare routine directly contradicts everything I know about skin and any science-based ideas about skincare.

Yes, lots of Korean women have beautiful skin. But it's not because their bathrooms are filled with expensive skincare products. It's probably largely genetic and also behavioural as these women generally avoid the sun. I am sure some of the products are lovely to use and many people swear by this type of regime to keep them happy with their skin, but to me it sounds like a classic Big Skincare marketing and sales tool. Don't forget that a ten-step skincare routine requires the purchase of *at least* ten products. What a fantastic business model!

The bottom line: Save your money. Korean skincare products are not magic and Korean women have genetics to thank for their lovely smooth skin (and perhaps their local consultant dermatologists . . .).

JADE ROLLERS

The jade face roller is touted as a panacea for skin issues: it can apparently reduce under-eye dark circles, shrink pores, minimise fine lines and wrinkles, and potentially lots of other things as well. But does it do anything beneficial? (And isn't this another example of skincare cultural appropriation?)

Let's use some common sense here . . . Do you think pressing a cold spoon to your face does anything beneficial to your skin? No, right? So, what is magical about a face roller made of stone? Zilch. Nada. Nothing. And there is definitely no scientific evidence for any of these jade roller claims.

Jade rollers are inexpensive and they aren't harmful to the skin, so if you like them, go for it. But they are in no way going to give you any long-term skincare benefits. Save your pennies and your hope – this is yet another marketing gimmick created by Big Skincare.

SERUMS

A serum is just another skincare product that has been added to the skincare world to get you to buy more stuff. No one 'needs' to use a serum or will in any way benefit from 'layering' various serums under their moisturisers or make-up. A serum is simply a more watery version of a 'moisturiser' but without any of the 'moisturising' components (like humectants or occlusives) of a proper emollient. Do you need a hyaluronic acid (HA) serum or a vitamin C serum or any other type of serum? Absolutely not. Keep your skincare simple, inexpensive and effective and don't put your hope in the next magic 'serum' to correct any skin concern you may have.

FACE MASKS

Face masks can be made of a multitude of substances, including clay and exotic-sounding ingredients. Sheet masks are face-shaped sheets that are 'soaked' in various types of serums like HA and vitamins. The idea is to 'nourish' the skin and the sheet itself apparently aids 'absorption' of all these nourishing compounds into the skin.

Are they 'effective' at 'nourishing' the skin? Don't waste your time or money. Masks of any kind are not helpful for skin; if anything, they give a short-term hydrating effect that can make the skin look smoother and therefore temporarily 'brighter', but the key concept here is 'temporary'. These sheet masks should not be viewed as treatments for actual skin problems.

The bottom line: If you like sheet masks or any type of mask and want to spend money on them, go for it. But don't expect them to impart long-lasting change to your skin.

LED LIGHT MASKS

There have only been a handful of studies looking at the effects of at-home LED masks, which is perhaps surprising considering their extortionate retail price points. The most recent one was published in 2020.[2] The objective of the study was to see if the masks improved the visible signs of skin ageing – 'facial rejuvenation' – by looking at changes in skin elasticity, hydration, texture and wrinkles over eight weeks. And the results? There were no significant differences at any point in the eight weeks in changes in skin hydration, wrinkles, roughness or smoothness of the skin. This means that any changes observed on the LED-treated side were the same on the non-treated side.

Oddly, the only thing that did change more significantly on the LED side and was statistically significant was an improvement in skin elasticity (this was tested using a device that is like a suction cup). If you really look at the numbers, you see that the control group had a significant improvement in skin elasticity from baseline at week six only, but not at week eight, while the LED group had a significant improvement at weeks six and eight only and the difference between the LED and the control group was significant at weeks six and eight. Though this study is probably a better one than its predecessors in terms of methodology and design, it definitely does not provide any evidence that these at-home LED masks are worth your hard-earned money or time.

The bottom line: At-home LED light masks for anti-ageing are a scam – don't buy one!

COLLAGEN AND OTHER SKIN SUPPLEMENTS

You do not need to take a skin-specific supplement or collagen supplement – ever – but these types of 'skin' supplements are probably not harmful. I would not be able to suggest that my patients spend money on these sorts of supplements as evidence for a true skin benefit to justify the cost is just not there.

To say that the published scientific literature on skin supplements is confusing is quite an understatement. This area is rife with poor-quality trials, dodgy methodology and small patient numbers, all sponsored or paid for by the companies that make the products. Obviously, these companies have a massive financial interest in getting people to use these products – the global collagen market is estimated to reach a value of nearly $4.6 billion by 2023![3]

Ingested nutrients don't generally translate into your body storing and utilising said nutrient in a productive or beneficial way. As we saw in Chapter 1, collagen is the most abundant protein in the body – it is not only in the skin but also in the connective tissue in the joints and in the lining of the digestive tract. It's basically everywhere. Your body makes all the collagen it needs from the amino acids that you eat.

When you ingest collagen – or any protein – your digestive system breaks it down and absorbs the amino acids. There is no guarantee that the collagen from your fancy £5 gold capsules are, after being absorbed, directly heading to your skin to rebuild your dermal collagen structure, leaving you with plumped-up skin. That is just not logical.

The bottom line: Don't bother with skin or collagen supplements. Just eat a balanced diet. Your wallet will thank you.

FACE YOGA

No one needs to do face yoga or 'facial exercises'.

Proponents of facial yoga refer to a study published in *JAMA Dermatology* in 2018 as 'evidence' that facial yoga 'works'.[4] Let's have a quick look at this evidence. This was a 'research letter' that wanted to examine if doing facial exercises could 'rejuvenate' the ageing face by 'inducing underlying muscle growth'. The authors call this a 'clinical trial' though the methodology used would not really classify this as a true clinical trial. But, for the sake of discussion, let's pretend that it is.

The study cohort consisted of 22 females aged 40–65 and they received 2 live 90-minute 'muscle-resistant facial exercise training sessions'. There was no blinding in the study; in other words, all participants – including the investigators – knew what product was being used. The participants then had to do daily 30-minute exercise sessions for 8 weeks, then on alternate days from weeks 9–20. Of the 22 people enrolled, only 16 completed the study.

The only 'positive' or mildly statistically significant outcome after 20 weeks was an increase in upper cheek and lower cheek 'fullness'. Whether this was due to muscle growth or not is unclear, though the authors attributed it to 'exercise-actuated hypertrophy of cheek and other muscles'. The mean average age appearance of the participants apparently decreased by two years.

Does this provide enough evidence to justify you paying a monthly subscription and committing 30 minutes a week to this, in the name of improving the appearance of your ageing face? Certainly not.

But can facial yoga or facial exercise be harmful? Yes it can, because wrinkles are partly due to chronic use of facial muscles over time (botulinum toxin – such as Botox – works to reduce wrinkles by stopping you from using the underlying muscle that is moving the skin). If you relax your forehead (frontalis) muscle, you won't be able to crease the skin overlying it, hence no wrinkles. But if you continue to move your face, you continue to crease the skin and, with time, those creases become deeper and more visible. This is the natural progression of wrinkles. So, if you want to stop that frown line between your eyebrows from becoming more prominent, you can do two things: stop frowning (which may not work for everyone, especially those with small children or dogs) or inject neurotoxin into those muscles to stop them from moving (see page 208). Moving the muscles more via facial exercises or facial yoga certainly will not help diminish those lines.

'COSMECEUTICALS' AND 'MEDICAL-GRADE SKINCARE'

According to the FDA, the term 'cosmeceutical' has no meaning under law. The skincare industry uses this word in reference to cosmetic products that they believe have 'medicinal' or 'drug-like' effects on the skin. Cosmetics are intended to beautify, alter the appearance of or cleanse the skin only; they are not meant to affect the skin's structure or function.

The word 'cosmeceutical' was first used by Dr Albert Kligman in 1984. But in 2000, he wrote, 'the term cosmeceutical has no legal status. Its prominence is due to its operational usefulness'.[5] Kligman had a love–hate relationship with this concept. On the one hand, he knew that some 'cosmetics', like salicylic acid, can be quite useful in the treatment of acne vulgaris, for example. He also knew that the idea that a cosmetic product could have a drug-like effect would be abused by the skincare industry for financial gain.

And over 20 years later, nothing much has changed, except the 'science' used to back up skincare claims has become more complex and the entire industry is worth billions of pounds. 'Medical-grade skincare' also doesn't have any real meaning: these are usually just regular cosmetic skincare products laced with exotic ingredients sold 'exclusively' at certain doctor's offices or 'medispas'. Stay away from these – they are horrendously overpriced and not unique in any way.

One way to think about it is that cosmetic skincare (this includes products labelled as cosmeceuticals or 'medical-grade skincare') refers to all skincare products that are not prescribed by a doctor. Now, this definition is not entirely accurate anymore because some licensed medicines are now available over the counter (but usually you must ask for them from the pharmacist). And dermatologists and GPs often do prescribe moisturisers and cleansers as part of treatment plans for patients with specific skin diseases. Perhaps a better definition of cosmetic skincare is anything that does not contain a medicine licensed for a specific condition. In fact, there are very few topical medicines used in normal dermatology practice; there are many more varieties of lotions and potions marketed and sold by Big Skincare. In dermatology practice, we stick to evidence-based topical medicines and that includes steroids, tacrolimus, tretinoin, hydroquinone, azelaic acid, ivermectin, topical antibiotics, vitamin D analogues and a handful of others.

These are true 'active' ingredients and have a vast amount of clinical data underlying their efficacy and safety in treating the specific condition they are licensed for. Cosmetic skincare, therefore, refers to anything that does not include one of these specific, targeted medicines and/or is not prescribed by a doctor. Most of these products are geared towards 'anti-ageing' or acne treatment.

Dermatologists use over-the-counter skincare products

alongside prescribed topical therapy (as adjuvants). The cosmetic skincare product is not the treatment. A doctor does not prescribe moisturiser alone to treat active eczema; if you have ever had active eczema, you would know that you can moisturise a hundred times a day, but the eczema doesn't get much better. It is the same with melasma (patches of brown pigmentation on the face) or acne. We have fantastic skin treatments for specific skin diseases available to patients as well as oral medications (tablets or capsules). You can't treat acne or melasma with a three-step skincare regime in the same way that you can't treat cancer by drinking kale juice and eating a low-carb diet; it might help you feel better or make you feel like you are doing something good for yourself, but, when it comes down to it, the treatment is the medicine.

I know what you are thinking: 'But what about vitamin C? What about HA, glycolic acid or niacinamide? Aren't these active ingredients too?' I define an active ingredient as something with a legitimate evidence base to prove that application of the topical in the *prescribed* dose causes a physiological change in the skin. But we need to be very careful here when looking at the evidence – most studies in modern-day 'skincare' are fully sponsored by the company that makes the product. And that fact alone introduces a huge amount of bias (see page 5).

What this means is that cosmetic skincare products are not regulated – as in, the company manufacturing and selling them does not need to provide any evidence that these products actually do anything useful for skin. The only thing that is regulated is how the companies are allowed to advertise what their products do, but often these rules have loopholes that are easily manipulated by clever marketing people.

When patients see an improvement in their skin condition or the overall appearance of their skin (like more 'glow' or softer skin texture) from using a cosmetic skincare regime, I always remind them that it is the act of consistently following a skincare regime (no matter how basic) that had an effect, not that specific skincare regime or using a particular product range or brand.

Of course, the choice of what product or products you choose to use (if any) really comes down to personal preference and budget. What I always say to my patients is 'buy what you like and can afford'. If you like using eye cream and layering on serums or love your Korean ten-step regime, and you don't have any major facial skin problems that need appropriate management, then go for it. In the same way that some people collect fancy cars or expensive shoes, some people collect skincare. But don't expect it to halt the ageing process or reverse any actual skin diseases you may currently have. Because, regardless of what the product packaging is telling you, this is a cosmetic skincare product and has no true evidence base for treating skin disease or even preventing wrinkles behind it.

If you want to use skincare that lives up to its claims, let's move on to Part 3.

PART 3

Unravelling Big Skincare Ingredient Claims

Perfect skin has become the thinking woman's quest. It's normal today for people in certain circles to brag about spending most of their paycheck on serums. The latest skincare trends have a reassuring scientific cast: peptides, acids, solutions, and other things with clinical suffixes that are typically sold in small quantities for large amounts of money.

But all of this is a scam . . .

Krithika Varagur, www.theoutline.com[1]

It is crucial to remember that 'cosmeceutical' or cosmetic skincare products are *not* claiming to affect the structure and function of the skin; if they did, they would need to be classified as drugs. Big Skincare skirts around this issue by using very careful marketing statements and claims that the advertising standards agencies and drug regulatory bodies cannot criticise. But the average consumer will almost certainly not pick up on the subtle difference between the statements 'may improve the appearance of fine lines' and 'may improve fine lines'. The first is a cosmetic skincare claim; the second a drug claim.

In practice, it is the *claims* made for the product that dictate whether it is a cosmetic or a drug, not necessarily the components.[2] In theory, it is possible for a product to be classified as a cosmetic *and* a drug, depending on its intended use. If the intended use is simply to enhance appearance, the product is classified as a cosmetic. If the intended use is to treat a disease, it is a drug.

So how do you go about trying to unravel the claims made by Big Skincare? 'With difficulty' is the answer! When I became a consultant dermatologist and started working in the private sector, I realised that patients have far more questions about cosmetic skincare products than anything else. In my clinical practice, on social media, from friends, family or any random people I meet, the minute they find out I am a dermatologist I get quizzed on the efficacy of claims of cosmetic products. It literally never ends.

When faced with these questions, I must make sure my answers and critical appraisal are clinically and scientifically sound. This requires me to use not only my knowledge of the structure and function of human skin in both health and disease, but also my knowledge of pharmacology, cellular biology, immunology and chemistry. And then I use my clinical experience to put it all together and make it relevant to my patients.

Usually (but not always), cosmetic products have a 'star' ingredient that is meant to do all the magic and consumers often think of skincare products in terms of 'active ingredients'. I use a three-question system to evaluate if a product or ingredient will do what it is claiming to do. I have adapted this from the work of Dr Douglas Kligman, a dermatologist in Pennsylvania.[3]

1. Can the active ingredient pass through the stratum corneum and get to the target cell or structure in the skin in the right amount or concentration necessary to have its intended effect?

2. Is there a specific cell or tissue in human skin that the active ingredient specifically targets in order to exert or achieve its intended effect?

3. Are there 'good-quality' clinical trials, as judged by the standards of the FDA or MHRA, to substantiate the active ingredients efficacy claims? 'Good quality' means trials that are published in peer-reviewed journals, that are double-blind and placebo-controlled as well as having statistically significant findings.

SKINTELLIGENT FACT:

How drugs are approved

Drugs need approval from the government of the country where they will be prescribed by doctors to be allowed to be prescribed as medicines. FDA stands for 'Food and Drug Administration' and is the American body that does this. In the UK, it's the MHRA (Medicines and Healthcare Products Regulatory Agency) and in Europe it's the EMA (European Medicines Agency). To get approval, a drug needs to be proven to fix a problem and generally it needs to show this by providing evidence in at least two well-designed, randomised, placebo-controlled trials.

How ingredients get into the skin

Let's start with the first question. How do ingredients penetrate the stratum corneum? It's meant to be a barrier, right? Remember that in between the corneoctyes are the winding, fat-filled pathways that allow for the flow (passive diffusion) of molecules from the outside in (see page 41).[4] The permeability of the stratum corneum can also be enhanced by a variety of chemical and physical techniques, including simple occlusion (covering it with a protective seal).

There are four primary ways in which molecules can penetrate the stratum corneum:[5]

1. Intercellular: via the fat-filled pathway between the corneocytes.
2. Transcellular: through the corneocyte.
3. Intrafollicular: via the hair follicle.
4. Pore: via the opening of a sweat gland on the skin surface.

PATHWAYS OF PENETRATION THROUGH THE SKIN

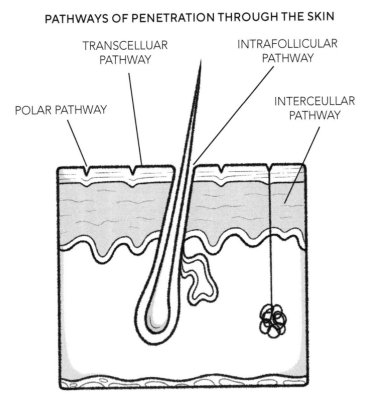

TRANSCELLUAR PATHWAY

INTRAFOLLICULAR PATHWAY

POLAR PATHWAY

INTERCEULLAR PATHWAY

There are hydrophilic (water-loving) channels in between the lipid bilayers between the corneoctyes, but the stratum corneum is generally hydrophobic (water-repelling) so fat-soluble molecules generally get through more easily than water-soluble ones. Water-soluble molecules can penetrate the skin via the openings of sweat glands and hair follicles, though the total surface area of these openings is only 0.1 per cent of the total skin surface area, making it probably insignificant. The only way to bypass the properties of the stratum corneum is to physically disrupt it, like with using adhesive tape to strip off the corneal layer.[6]

The widest gap between the intercellular lipids measures only 0.013μm and that's how 90 per cent of molecules penetrate the skin. A molecule of 500 dalton is the maximum mass that allows penetration in the stratum corneum (see 'The 500 dalton rule' below).

SKINTELLIGENT FACT:

The 500 dalton rule

A dalton is a unit used to measure the weight of proteins in chemistry or physics. It is analogous to kilograms or pounds, which are the units used to measure how heavy something is – its mass.

There are a variety of different active molecules used in dermatology to treat skin disease, and they all have a molecular weight less than 500 dalton. This includes terbinafine (291 – an antifungal) and all topical steroids (around 400), as well as medicines used via transdermal drug delivery systems (patches) like nicotine (162), oestradiol (272) and testosterone (288).

The molecular weights (in dalton) of the specific ingredients discussed in this section are as follows:

- Retinoic acid: 300
- Hydroquinone: 110
- Ascorbic acid (vitamin C): 176
- Glycolic acid: 76
- Salicylic acid: 138
- Azelaic acid: 188
- Copper peptides: 404
- Hyaluronic acid: 4,000–8,000,000
- Bakuchiol: 256
- Niacinamide: 122

Arguments against the 500 dalton rule are that via the appropriate formulation or even with the use of penetration enhancers, higher molecular weight substances can conceivably penetrate the stratum corneum. Though neither of these statements has been proven, this is one way Big Skincare can market products, such as hyaluronic acid, which, as you can see, is way too big to penetrate the stratum corneum.[7]

Remember that not all ingredients need to enter the skin to do something – often they can just do something by sitting on top of it. Cosmetic skincare products – by virtue of being cosmetic and intended to temporarily enhance the appearance of the skin – do not penetrate the epidermis or dermis. But this does not necessarily mean the product is ineffective because, as already discussed in relation to moisturisers and sunscreen, these products can still serve to protect the stratum corneum and enable it to achieve its function as the body's first and essential barrier (see page 13).

How ingredients affect the skin

Let's say an ingredient can penetrate the stratum corneum, and it can penetrate to the depth required and in the concentration necessary to exert some type of biological effect. The next step, then, is how does the ingredient exert its effect? Most medicines or active drugs that create biologic change do this by changing how a cell functions. This can happen through inhibiting or activating an enzyme, acting on a receptor in or on the cell to stimulate a chemical signal or even activating a gene.

For example, vitamin K is an important cofactor in enzyme reactions in the liver as part of blood clotting. Basically, you need vitamin K to clot blood. Bruising happens after trauma to the skin because red blood cells come out of the blood vessels in the skin and accumulate in the dermis. Creams with vitamin K in them are sold as helpful for speeding up the resolution of bruises. Vitamin K weighs 450 dalton so it can penetrate the skin – but what does it do when it gets there? What happens in the skin to speed up the clearance of the bruise? A bruise is by definition already clotted blood (the blood isn't flowing), so even if vitamin K got to the bruise it would not do anything to help the bruise go away more quickly.

The bottom line: Any ingredient applied to the skin needs to be able to exert its effect through reaching the intended target and being able to do something there.

HOW WE KNOW THE INGREDIENT 'WORKS'

The major issue here is that over the past 20 or so years so many trials have suffered from extreme bias; as we've seen, Big Skincare is worth billions of pounds so there are a lot of stakeholders involved. Unfortunately, many of these stakeholders are scientists and doctors (including dermatologists) who have a vested financial interest in selling expensive cosmetic products.

We know that 'spin' happens in skincare-related scientific papers. Spin occurs when the conclusions drawn by the authors don't match what the results of the trial actually show; in other words, reporting that distorts the interpretation of results. That's why just reading the abstract and/or conclusion of a scientific paper can be very misleading. Unfortunately, that is what many people do and it leads to lots of incorrect headlines in beauty publications, online and in the media. People then purchase those products because they believe the 'science'.

A group of dermatologists performed a systematic review of placebo-controlled double-blind clinical trials of the topical treatment of photoaged skin to identify if spin was used and what kind. They searched the literature and only uncovered 20 relatively 'high-quality' trials (out of a possible 951 that fit the initial search criteria). What they found was quite extraordinary – and very worrying.[8] All the studies had conclusions that were not in keeping with what the results actually showed and, importantly, all the articles reviewed concluded that the topical application of the test products showed promise in the treatment of photoaged skin. At least 16 out of the 20 papers were sponsored by the manufacturer of the test product and all of them were trials of cosmetic skincare products – not medicines or prescription topical treatments.[9]

The bottom line: Don't trust Big Skincare, even if the advertisement quotes a published scientific paper. These are 'marketing' clinical trials – they are intended to increase sales, not provide useful scientific information.

If you are struggling with a skin condition, you may be vulnerable and easily manipulated into purchasing cosmetic skincare products with the hope of a 'quick fix'. And Big Skincare is more than happy to supply you with an abundance of seemingly effective options that generally have no evidence of efficacy. Though these products might not harm your skin (and not help either), they may certainly harm your mental health or general well-being, if you have spent more money and are disappointed that your skin problem still isn't under control.

In the chapters that follow I am going to carry out an in-depth analysis of specific, 'trendy' or controversial ingredients found in modern skincare, some of which Big Skincare makes claims about, and uncover the truth.

7

Vitamin A

When it comes to the discussion of vitamin A, I have noticed – online, with my own clients and in the media – that a lot of confusion stems from the terminology used. If we are going to have a sensible discussion, we all need to be on the same page with our vocabulary.

Here are the definitions for some of the most commonly used words in the discussion of vitamin A:

- Retinoid: umbrella term encompassing a family of chemical compounds that are natural or synthetic vitamin A derivatives that share structural and functional similarity with vitamin A; all the vitamin A derivatives fall under this term. In my clinical practice, the term 'retinoid' is used to specifically refer to retinoic acid.
- Retinoic acid: the biologically active retinoid that acts on specific retinoic acid receptors throughout human tissue. There are many synthetic versions of retinoic acid that are used for a variety of conditions, both orally and topically.
- Retinol: the main circulating form of vitamin A that requires conversion to the active retinoic acid to have a biological effect on tissues. This term is often used to refer to vitamin A derivatives used as ingredients in over-the-counter non-prescription cosmetic skincare products that are not classified as medicines.
- Tretinoin: a synthetic version of biologically active retinoic acid that is the most investigated retinoid in the treatment

of intrinsically and photoaged skin. In many countries, tretinoin is only available on prescription. Brand names for tretinoin include, but are not limited to: Acretin, Renova, Retin-A, Avita, Atralin, Retin-A Micro and Avage.

- Adapalene: a third-generation (newer) retinoid that is specifically licensed for the treatment of acne. It selectively binds the retinoic acid receptors beta and gamma receptors. Brand names include Differin and Adaferin.

- Tazarotene: a third-generation (newer) retinoid that is licensed for the treatment of psoriasis, acne and photodamage. It selectively binds to retinoic acid beta and gamma. Brand names include Tazorac, Avage and Zorac.

I generally prescribe tretinoin, so in this book and in my day-to-day practice I use the terms 'tretinoin', 'retinoid' and 'retinoic acid' interchangeably, as all referring to the same thing. If I want to speak about one of the other retinoids, like adapalene, I will refer to it as such.

RETINOIC ACID

Both the basic science and clinical dermatological literature have shown beyond a doubt that **retinoic acid can have profound effects on both the dermis and epidermis**. The basic biochemistry, molecular biology and pharmacology of retinoic acid – the FDA-approved drug – are well-established. Since 1969, retinoic acid has been used to treat acne and it works mainly by 'unsticking' the cells lining the hair follicles, which are the main cause of comedones (see page 63). Over years it was observed that patients treated with topical retinoic acid (tretinoin) for acne often developed smoother, less wrinkled skin. The effects of retinoic acid on ageing and photoaged skin were therefore studied and culminated in commercialisation and FDA approval for the use of tretinoin in the treatment of fine lines.[1]

Tretinoin

Tretinoin was the first and still the only topical treatment shown to improve the appearance of photoaged human skin through hundreds of robust clinical trials. It's the real deal. For example, one study showed an 80 per cent increase in the quantity of collagen building blocks in the dermis after 12 months of daily use of topical tretinoin (0.1 per cent), which led to the remodelling of about 6 per cent of the mature collagen network, causing a clinical improvement in the appearance of photodamaged skin.[2]

When tretinoin is used continuously for at least a few months, the following changes occur in the skin (these are changes you would see if your treated skin was biopsied and compared to your 'untreated' skin):

- replacement of a thinning (atrophic) epidermis with one composed of new, healthy cells
- the elimination of abnormal-looking (atypical) keratinocytes (skin cells) in the epidermis
- clearance of sun-damaged skin cells ('actinic keratosis')
- new collagen formation in the papillary (upper) dermis
- new blood vessels in the dermis
- exfoliation of shed but not desquamated (removed from the skin) skin cells in the hair follicles

The bottom line: These types of studies show that topical tretinoin is capable of partly reversing some of the structural damage due to ageing and sun exposure.[3] But don't get actual retinoic acid (tretinoin) confused with over-the-counter, cosmetic vitamin A derivatives, which are not classified as medicines and are not the same thing. These types of derivatives are found in many skincare products with the following names: retinol, retinaldehyde, retinal, retinyl esters, retinyl palmitate, retinyl propionate, retinyl retinoate and retinyl N-formyl aspartamate.

SKINTELLIGENT FACT:

How retinoic acid works

Retinoic acid changes skin by modifying or altering the ways the cell differentiates, through a direct action on DNA. There are retinoic acid receptors on the surface of keratinocytes (see page 21). In this way, it leads to thickening of the epidermis, stimulating the fibroblasts to produce more collagen and stopping collagen from being broken down by reducing the activity of the enzymes that work to break down collagen.[4]

VITAMIN A AND AGEING

Renova is an FDA-approved tretinoin cream (it's not yet available in the UK) for the 'mitigation of fine facial wrinkles in patients who use comprehensive skincare and sunlight avoidance programs'.[5] The package insert for the product states: 'Renova does not eliminate wrinkles, repair sun-damaged skin, reverse photoaging or restore more youthful or younger skin.'[6] Five clinical trials with a total of 279 participants were performed by the pharma company to get FDA approval: 10.4 per cent of the participants who used tretinoin and sunscreen had a moderate improvement in fine wrinkling, compared with 3 per cent of those who only used sunscreen.[7] That means 90 per cent of participants saw less than moderate or no improvement in fine wrinkling.

We are quite used to seeing skincare products advertised with claims like '8 out of 10 women saw a dramatic improvement in the appearance of their crow's feet after 12 weeks of use.' So 10.4 per cent of 279 people seeing only a 'moderate' improvement in fine lines looks, well, not great. And this is just one example. There are several other retinoic acids that have been FDA approved as 'anti-fine-wrinkle-only' creams and the clinical trial findings are similar. If it's true that the 'gold-standard' prescription anti-ageing cream isn't even that great at improving the signs of ageing, where does that leave over-the-counter vitamin A derivative products? Not worth the money, that's for sure!

Skincare retailers sell a plethora of retinol-containing products – ranging from serums and moisturisers to masks and eye creams – with prices ranging from £4.20 for a 30-ml serum to £210 for a 50-ml cream (so most of these products are much more expensive than prescription tretinoin). I critically appraised the randomised, double-blind, vehicle-controlled trials of the use of over-the-counter vitamin A products in the treatment of facial skin ageing, to assess evidence for its efficacy, and found that nine trials fit the criteria.[8] Four of the trials showed no statistically significant differences between the vitamin A derivative product and vehicle. The remaining five trials provided weak evidence for the vitamin A derivative product potentially having a mild positive effect on fine facial skin wrinkle lines only. However, these five trials all had major issues with how they were performed (the method), which calls into question the validity of any positive results.

I concluded that, in the case of these vitamin A derivative products, the 'positive' trials were not done to inform clinical decision-making, but rather to serve as tools for advertising. Until at least one high-quality clinical trial of a vitamin A derivative product in the treatment of photoaged skin is published, there is very little, if any, trustworthy evidence to support the use of them to improve the appearance of aged skin.

SKINTELLIGENT TIP:

Cosmetic 'retinol' products are a waste of time and money

No one can sensibly argue that over-the-counter vitamin A derivative products are better or more effective than true retinoic acid, like tretinoin. When faced with skincare confusion, remember that this is a billion-pound industry; most people are not looking out for your skin or wallet's best interest and it's a business. Sadly, even doctors have fallen prey to this, which negatively affects the entire medical profession.

It is, however, important to note that **there is no other topical treatment – prescription, over-the-counter or cosmetic – that has more high-quality evidence to support its ability to even mildly lessen the appearance of fine lines than tretinoin**. Dr Albert Kligman pioneered the use of topical retinoic acid for anti-ageing and has written time and again about the use of tretinoin for the entire face, and he specifically mentions around the mouth, nose and eyes: 'To eradicate wrinkles around the eyes and mouth, we urge that the medicament be applied right up to the borders, while suggesting that the transient stinging and burning is a useful sign of adequate coverage. No harm is done when small amounts of tretinoin enter the eyes or lips.'[9] Tretinoin can, however, collect in the creases around your nose and eyes (the lower eyelid and where your smile lines – 'crow's feet' – are), therefore causing more irritation in those areas, so be careful that you apply only a small amount to these areas. Definitely avoid the upper eyelid for this reason.

SKINTELLIGENT TIP:

Listen to your mother

My mum turned 70 in 2020. She started using topical tretinoin when she was 30 (right after she had me!) at the suggestion of my dad (who is not a derm, but wishes he was – he's a neurologist).

My mum has never had Botox or fillers or a facelift. She's never had microneedling or a 'laser' facial. She never wears make-up aside from a red lipstick. She's never done anything to her face – quite literally – except use tretinoin religiously every-single-night. She now uses 0.1 per cent and a moisturiser from Neutrogena. She doesn't use a cleanser.

My mum loves to sunbathe and always has, but she uses sunscreen (just on her face though – you can lead a horse to water . . .). My mum has beautiful skin – it's like a plump apple.

Skincare wasn't something I grew up with; only when I started having skin issues in my teens did I force my mum to buy me expensive lotions and potions from Bloomingdale's. She very kindly went along with it.

I have now come full circle and I am doing pretty much the same skincare routine my mum has done for the past 40 years. And my own skin has never looked better. It just took me 15 years of medical school and dermatology training to get me there! I should have listened to my mother.

THE MOST COMMON QUESTIONS I GET ASKED ABOUT TOPICAL RETINOIDS

What is retinoid dermatitis?

Since the early 1980s, up to 92 per cent of subjects using tretinoin in various studies report what has been coined 'retinoid dermatitis' – the development of red, itchy, flaky skin at the site of application. In some patients, this is a serious limitation to the use of topical retinoids and it has also raised the question whether 'irritation' is the mechanism underlying the long-term positive repairing effects of treatment. In other words, if you don't get skin irritation from using topical retinoids then it must not be 'working'. To answer this question, a study was performed comparing the efficacy and irritation of two concentrations of tretinoin cream – 0.1 and 0.025 per cent. The treatments were used once daily for 48 weeks and there was no significant difference in the overall improvement in photoageing produced by the two concentrations, but 0.1 per cent tretinoin was significantly more irritating.[10]

So why does the irritation occur and what can you do about it?

No one really knows what causes retinoid dermatitis. One study suggests that it might be due, at least partially, to an 'overload' of the retinoic acid receptors when a large amount of retinoic acid suddenly goes into the skin and the excess retinoic acid that cannot bind to the receptors ends up just causing inflammation and irritation.[11]

When I am treating the signs of ageing skin, I generally start my patients on the lowest possible concentration of tretinoin – usually 0.025 per cent – and start them off by using it three times a week only for the first four weeks. If irritation occurs, I advise patients to stop using it until their skin is back to normal and then start again. It is important to apply the tretinoin to thoroughly dry skin to minimise irritation. I also suggest applying a bland emollient (like Vaseline) *before* the tretinoin at bedtime to further minimise irritation at the beginning of treatment. Studies show that doing this does not reduce the efficacy of the tretinoin, even in acne patients, but it does minimise the irritation.[12]

Do retinoids increase or decrease the sun sensitivity of skin?

If you are using a topical retinoid either for acne treatment or to combat the signs of ageing and photodamage, I am pretty sure you will have been warned that the treatment will make you more prone to burning in the sun, so you have to wear a sunscreen daily. But is this true? If it is, why and how does a topical retinoid do this?

There is a good amount of experimental evidence to show that **topical tretinoin not only prevents collagen in the skin from being damaged by sun exposure but also repairs already damaged collagen**. Studies show that pretreatment of sun-protected human skin with tretinoin can significantly reduce the damaging effects of UVB light on collagen in the dermis. There is also a possible additional way in which tretinoin may prevent photoageing: UV light seems to cause a 'functional' vitamin A deficiency in the skin, which might be one of the many ways in which UV light damages the skin. Pretreatment with tretinoin seems to prevent this from occurring (though it's much more complicated than this!). Paradoxically, it seems that retinoids also act as UV filters because their molecular side chains contain conjugated double bonds, which strongly absorb UV light.

In short, all this evidence suggests that topical retinoids have a 'sunscreen' effect. However, the stratum corneum is made more compact (which some people refer to as 'thinned') in the first few months of tretinoin therapy and, therefore, it is necessary to wear sunscreen to protect yourself from burning. This increased risk of burning goes away after about six months of continuous use in line with the stratum corneum no longer being compacted.[13]

Do you need to stop using tretinoin in the summertime or before you go on holiday?

Absolutely not – I would advise you to make sure you keep using it! Regardless of whether you are using a topical retinoid, you should *always* be vigilant about sun protection for so many reasons (and I know you know all of these – to prevent ageing, skin cancer, pigmentation, and so on), but also because you are using the topical retinoid to make your skin look better and reverse the signs of chronic sun exposure, the main one of which is the development of fine lines. Using an SPF50 (or more) and wearing a wide-brimmed hat (or staying out of the sun entirely) is going to support you in achieving your skincare goals, while going out in the sun (even with sunscreen on) could potentially set you back and reverse all the good work.

How long does it take to see results from topical retinoids?

For general skin rejuvenation and anti-ageing, you should start seeing an improvement in skin texture and fine lines within a few weeks of using a high-quality prescription retinoid; your skin should feel softer and smoother.

For comedones and acne, it takes a bit longer to see an improvement; retinoids work for acne by reducing the number of comedones, and this takes time. If your acne is mild, you will see an improvement more quickly, likely within 8–12 weeks. However, if your acne is severe it will take longer and I suggest that a retinoid alone isn't going to be enough. You should see a consultant dermatologist to discuss more potent treatment options (see page 277). A retinoid will always be the backbone of any acne treatment regime as well as long-term maintenance, so definitely keep using it even if you don't see results quickly. Achieving great skin is a marathon, not a sprint, and requires lifelong maintenance to keep it clear and looking good.

Do retinoids thin the skin?

No. As we've seen, during the first six months of daily use of tretinoin, biopsy studies show that the epidermis (top layer of the skin) gets thicker, primarily because one of the layers (the stratum granulosum) gets 'thicker' and the stratum corneum becomes more compact – which some people misinterpret as the skin getting 'thinner'. Therefore, skin is more susceptible to sunburn in the first six months of treatment.

With continued use, however, at 12 months, when examined under a microscope, all these changes revert to 'baseline'. Interestingly, any clinical improvement found in fine lines is still apparent even at this 12-month mark. This is a little bit of a conundrum because it appears that the changes we see under a microscope don't necessarily correlate with what is seen clinically (in real-life patients). Nevertheless, there is no evidence to suggest that retinoids 'thin the skin'.[14]

HOW TO USE A RETINOID WITH OTHER SKINCARE PRODUCTS

Just because you start using prescription skincare to deal with your primary skin concern, that doesn't mean you need to ditch your entire arsenal of favourite skincare products. A retinoid can be used at the same time as most of your other over-the-beauty-counter lotions and potions, taking into account a few simple 'rules' to make sure your retinoid still gets the spotlight.

Some basics: never exfoliate with a scrub – retinoids are very powerful exfoliators in their own right so you don't need to do anything extra. Plus scrubs and scrubbing can damage your delicate epidermis (that's the top layer of your skin) so are best avoided. In the same vein, consider stopping any acid products, whether in creams or toners. Again, retinoids are powerful exfoliators so if you use an acid product as well you might dry out your skin too much and cause redness, flaking and irritation, especially when you are just starting out. Also, avoid or be careful when getting hot treatments on your face, like waxing and lasers, because your skin will be more light- and heat-sensitive. Threading and electrolysis are great alternatives for facial hair removal (see page 251). In addition, only use your retinoid at night because the medicine gets degraded by sunlight:

1. Cleanse your skin using an oil cleanser, making sure to remove your make-up thoroughly. Pat your skin dry and allow it to dry completely (this should only take a few seconds).
2. Apply your prescribed treatment as per your doctor's directions.
3. Apply moisturiser – go for a greasy one (see page 80)!

If you find that your skin is getting excessively irritated or dry when using a retinoid, apply your moisturiser before you apply your retinoid.

When using a retinoid, you should use acid-based products, vitamin C and any of your other favourite products like serums in your morning skincare routine only. But beware that, even then, using different exfoliators can lead to redness and irritation, especially when you first start using a retinoid, so consider sticking to a simplified skincare routine when starting out. I always suggest that my patients, at least for the first few weeks of starting a prescribed product, stop all other skincare aside from a basic oil cleanser, greasy moisturiser and sunscreen.

The bottom line: Tretinoin is still the number one cream to improve the appearance of fine lines that develop as we get older.

8

Hydroquinone

Hydroquinone is the gold-standard prescription topical treatment for unwanted spots of pigmentation on the skin – like sun damage and sun freckles (solar lentigo), the dark spots that can appear from healed acne lesions (called post-inflammatory hyperpigmentation), as well as hormonal pigmentation like melasma (symmetrical brown patches on the face, often occurring during pregnancy – see page 221). It is so effective and so commonly prescribed that 30 million tubes of 2 per cent hydroquinone are produced worldwide per year, with about 50 per cent sold in the United States.[1]

In normal skin, melanocytes (the pigment-producing cells of the epidermis) convert the amino acid tyrosine into melanin via the enzyme tyrosinase. Hyperpigmentation occurs from an increase in melanin production and the most important risk factor for this is sunlight exposure and, in acne, it's due to inflammation.[2] Hydroquinone works by reversibly blocking tyrosinase and preventing melanin production. As the skin cells mature, the heavily pigmented skin cells are shed, and new skin cells are formed with less melanin. Hydroquinone works by gradually suppressing melanin pigment production – it does not 'bleach the skin', as commonly thought.[3]

Hydroquinone was first discovered to be a lightening agent in 1936. In the 1950s it was available over the counter as a sunscreen and in 1961 the first clinical trial of its use as a skin lightening agent was published and it became a medical product available commercially. In 2001, in EU countries, it became

HOW HYDROQUINONE WORKS TO SUPPRESS MELANIN PIGMENT PRODUCTION IN THE SKIN

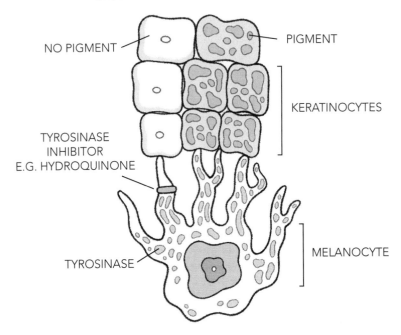

NO PIGMENT

PIGMENT

KERATINOCYTES

TYROSINASE INHIBITOR E.G. HYDROQUINONE

TYROSINASE

MELANOCYTE

no longer authorised for use in cosmetic skin lightening formulations, and only available on prescription.[4]

The EU restricted the use of hydroquinone-containing non-prescription anti-pigmentation creams based on case reports of side effects like worsening pigmentation (exogenous ochronosis) and excessive skin lightening (leukoderma) with the use of skin lighteners or photographic developers. Hydroquinone can still be found in nail polish systems and hair dyes in the EU.[5]

IS HYDROQUINONE SAFE TO USE?

Yes, it is. Hydroquinone is one of the longest-standing and most effective topical treatments we have in dermatology, with a massive amount of high-quality safety and efficacy data to support its use.[6]

There are, however, persistent concerns in the media and on the internet about its safety, with the two main ones being about exogenous ochronosis and cancer.

Hydroquinone and exogeneous ochronosis

Exogenous ochronosis is a paradoxical increase in pigmentation. It is thought to occur with prolonged application of hydroquinone combined with chronic sun exposure of the treated areas. This may cause melanocytes to pass down to the papillary (upper) dermis and be taken up by the fibroblast cells. They are then excreted by the fibroblasts as an altered fibre, which is deposited in the dermis and appears on sun-exposed parts of the skin as a blue-grey pigmentation.[7]

In a review of the literature from 1966 to 2007 for studies involving the use of hydroquinone in a clinical setting, total patient exposure was over 20,000 and duration of use went up to 240 months, with hydroquinone concentrations ranging from 1 to 30 per cent. In none of these studies was exogeneous ochronosis reported.[8] During this same period, there were only 22 cases of exogeneous ochronosis reported in the United States, 21 of which were associated with the use of 1–2 per cent hydroquinone and one of them from 4 per cent, with duration of use being years.[9] As you can see, exogeneous ochronosis is exceptionally rare; it is estimated that there is one case of exogenous ochronosis for every 300–450 million tubes of hydroquinone sold in the United States.

In the trials for FDA approval of Tri-Luma (a commercially available treatment containing hydroquinone, tretinoin and a mild topical steroid, licensed for the treatment of melasma), there were approximately 300 patients who had a cumulative use of Tri-Luma cream of more than six months. Some patients had continuous use for up to 12 months. No patient developed exogenous ochronosis. The most common adverse effects of Tri-Luma were skin redness, peeling, burning, dryness and itchiness. Subjects who had cumulative treatment of melasma with Tri-Luma cream for six months showed a similar pattern of adverse events as in eight-week studies.[10]

Does hydroquinone cause cancer?

No, it does not. There are numerous studies looking at human exposure to hydroquinone and there has not been a single cancer reported. There are some extreme studies out there too – like one in which 17 people ingested 300mg of hydroquinone per day for 30 months without developing any health problems, and another that looked at 879 people exposed to hydroquinone via skin contact while working in a hydroquinone production factory over a 50-year period. They found no adverse health impacts or evidence of cancer due to hydroquinone exposure in this population – the study population's health outcomes were actually better than those of the non-exposed control subjects. Indeed, hydroquinone is normally found in the blood and urine of humans who do not use it on their skin at all because it is found in bread, fruit, coffee and red wine.[11]

THE MOST COMMON QUESTIONS I GET ASKED ABOUT HYDROQUINONE

Does hydroquinone cause rebound pigmentation?

'Rebound' pigmentation is defined as pigmentation that comes back worse after stopping the treatment than it was before the treatment was started. This has never been reported in clinical trials using hydroquinone in the topical treatment of melasma or hyperpigmentation.[12]

Does hydroquinone need to be cycled every three months?

I have been prescribing hydroquinone in combination with tretinoin for years to effectively and safely treat facial pigmentation problems. One thing I am asked by patients is whether the treatment needs to be 'cycled' or whether they need a treatment break every few months. In medicine, a treatment break is sometimes required for some medicines to allow the patient to recover from the treatment and its side effects (like with chemotherapy for cancer). In dermatology, if a topical treatment is working to clear a skin problem, the patient keeps using it until the skin is clear and then tapers off the treatment to move into a maintenance regime of perhaps using it only once or twice a week. We would cycle treatments (for example three weeks using it, followed by a three-week break) if the side effects of the treatment are uncomfortable for the patient, like itchiness or soreness.

Hydroquinone may cause mild irritation or discomfort, but usually not badly enough to require a treatment break. It also does not 'stop working' after a certain amount of time. It should be used continuously until the skin problem (in this case, pigmentation) has cleared sufficiently. There seems to be an idea propagated on the internet and by Big Skincare that hydroquinone can cause exogenous ochronosis when used beyond three months. As we've seen, this side effect is extraordinarily uncommon and is not related to a specific length of use.

The only reason I would 'cycle' hydroquinone, or start to, is when my patients have achieved clearance of their pigmentation but they need to use something to prevent a melasma flare-up, for example in the sunnier months. I also increase or decrease the hydroquinone strength based on how patients are doing; there is no set number of weeks or months – it is totally dependent on the clinical picture. Because I am treating a skin problem, not a number or day target, I treat what I see.

That's the beauty of dermatology: if it's not there and you can't see it, it doesn't need treatment.

SKINTELLIGENT TIP:

How to use hydroquinone to treat melasma and facial hyperpigmentation

Below are the evidence-based guidelines on how to use hydroquinone safely and effectively (always follow the advice of your prescribing doctor):

- 'Treatment breaks' are not necessary. Hydroquinone does not stop working the longer you use it since the melanin pathway that it impacts does not become 'resistant' to tyrosinase inhibition.
- It is not necessary to use hydroquinone in a 'pulsed' way or to cycle it.[13]
- Hydroquinone does not cause 'rebound' pigmentation.
- Hydroquinone can work for melanocytic pigmentation on the body, but it is not as effective as it is on the face.
- Hydroquinone should be combined with tretinoin and a mild potency steroid (in a triple formulation) to treat melasma.[14]
- Ideally, hydroquinone should be used twice a day to treat melasma optimally.[15]
- Using sunscreen every day properly is extremely important to help minimise the risk of worsening the pigmentation during treatment or causing it to recur after successful treatment.[16]

- If you are seeing improvement in your pigmentation after three months but you still want more improvement, it is perfectly acceptable to continue using your hydroquinone-containing prescription topically for more than three months, under your doctor's direct medical supervision.

Your prescribing consultant dermatologist will tell you how to use your treatment. You should not be asking for or taking advice about how to use your prescription medicine from anyone but them.

A sincere request to non-prescribers in the skincare community (this includes journalists, facialists, cosmetic chemists and anyone else who is not trained and legally allowed to prescribe prescription-only medicines): please stop giving advice to users of prescription treatments about how to use their treatment or how to manage any side effects experienced. Much of the 'advice' given by non-prescribers is incorrect and misleading. Unfortunately, these people also often have large social media platforms and therefore this misinformation becomes propagated, leading to further confusion and mistrust.

Let's all show some respect for these treatments and for those of us who have spent many years not only studying but also gaining years of clinical experience in order to guide our patients safely and effectively through their treatment. We need to put an end to the 'fake news' and misinformation that those without the appropriate credentials are stating as facts.

The bottom line: There is a lot of negative publicity about hydroquinone (as is the case with many prescription treatments) that has no evidence base and no logic behind it. I would suggest that much of the negative press is propagated by Big Skincare that sees the use of hydroquinone as a threat to the sale of their own (very expensive and generally ineffective) 'anti-pigment' cosmetic products.

9

Vitamin C

Topical vitamins are big business in skincare. Let's step back for a second to look at some basic facts about vitamins. First, vitamins are organic substances that humans generally cannot make so they need to be ingested (usually in food). Vitamins are cofactors for enzyme reactions. Think of a cofactor as a 'helper' molecule. Enzymes are small protein molecules that allow two things (called 'substrates') to combine and form something new or to cause some sort of chemical reaction between two things – cofactors 'help' the enzyme do this more efficiently.

We mainly know about vitamins necessary for physical health when the vitamin has been severely depleted and causes disease. Probably the best-known example of this is scurvy, which is the name for vitamin C deficiency. Vitamin C (ascorbic acid) is a cofactor in several enzymatic reactions and is required for making collagen throughout the body, including in blood vessel walls, as well as for the absorption of iron in the gut and the metabolism of cholesterol. If you do not ingest vitamin C for at least three months, symptoms of scurvy will develop, which include bleeding sores, loss of teeth and anaemia. Thankfully, scurvy is extremely rare in the modern world – the last documented major 'outbreak' was during the war in Afghanistan in 2002.[1]

So why are topical vitamin C products so popular? That's a great question and one you have almost certainly thought about when faced with whether to purchase a £150, 30-ml bottle of vitamin C 'serum'. The studies and the marketing are extremely convincing – and it all comes down to the antioxidant effect.

UNDERSTANDING ANTIOXIDANTS

Before we delve into whether topical antioxidants really work to protect skin from oxidation, it's time for some basic science . . . The cells in our body use oxygen to generate energy. That energy is known as adenosine triphosphate (ATP) and is made by the mitochondria (the powerhouse of cells) in each and every cell in our body. When ATP is made via oxygen, free radicals are produced as a by-product and they are referred to as reactive oxygen species (ROS) and reactive nitrogen species (RNS). Free radicals are highly unstable molecules that have electrons readily available to react with various things in the body like lipids, proteins and DNA.[2]

Not all free radicals are bad though; at a low or moderate level, ROS and RNS have beneficial effects on cellular responses and immune function.[3] But at high concentrations – having too many free radicals – they can generate what is referred to as 'oxidative stress', which can damage cell structures and is known to play a role in the development of many chronic diseases such as arthritis and cardiovascular disease.

The body does have ways to balance the oxidative stress and these balancing agents are called antioxidants. They can be made in the body or supplied via food. They 'scavenge' the free radicals, thus preventing them from causing damage or repairing damage caused by ROS and RNS. The ones made in the body are called endogenous and include glutathione, lipoic acid, L-arginine, uric acid, bilirubin and transferrin. Nutrient antioxidants cannot be produced in the body and must be provided via food, and these include vitamin E, vitamin C and omega-3 and omega-6 fatty acids.

Free radicals can be produced both endogenously (in your body) and exogenously (from external sources). Inflammation, mental stress, excessive exercise, cancer, infection and just getting older are all ways free radicals are generated endogenously. Exogenous sources include pollution, cigarette smoke, alcohol, radiation and certain drugs.[4]

It is generally accepted that oxidative stress is part of the ageing process, but oral supplementation with exogenous nutrient antioxidants doesn't seem to be the answer. This applies to vitamin C, which, as most of you will know, also acts as an antioxidant. Though the positive effects seem to be that it may reduce the risk of certain cancers, higher doses (2,000mg or more per day) are controversial because there is some evidence to suggest it can be 'pro-oxidant' or carcinogenic.[5]

Topical antioxidants

Now back to skin ... UV light from the sun generates free radicals in the skin, which results in tissue damage and an inflammatory response (if extreme, this is classic 'sunburn'). Human skin contains endogenous (already found in the skin) antioxidants including glutathione and uric acid. The idea here is that by applying antioxidants topically to the skin, they will work by 'scavenging' the free radicals and, in theory, supplying excess levels above the endogenous levels is beneficial to skin. So how likely is it that applying topical antioxidants to the skin can prevent further photodamage from occurring?

Not very likely. The negative effects of UV light on skin happen in real time so the antioxidant must be present continuously in or on the skin at the correct concentration without being inactivated. So, if topical vitamins are meant to work as photoprotectants, they need to undergo the same type of vigorous real-life testing as sunscreens. More research is needed in this area.

There is a plethora of vitamin-C-containing products on the

market today. However, vitamin C is incredibly unstable as a molecule as it oxidises rapidly. If we want vitamin C to work as a photoprotector via its antioxidant capability, we must ask how often it needs to be applied to the skin. Would it be valuable or useful to increase epidermal concentrations of vitamin C? The ability of vitamin C to penetrate the skin is an important consideration here.

Vitamin C is a water-soluble and charged molecule and is repelled by the physical barrier of the cells of the epidermis. It is only when the pH level is below 3 and vitamin C is present as ascorbic acid in sufficient concentration that some penetration of the topical product occurs, but whether this results in increased levels in the stratum corneum, the viable epidermis or the dermis is unknown.[6] Added to that, it is not going to be present in any cosmetic formulation in sufficient concentration or in proper chemical form to act as a physiologic antioxidant, even if it is just sitting on the skin surface.[7]

Topically applied vitamin C probably does not reach the dermis in any significant concentration, so will it still be able to prevent some of the negative effects of UVA damage on elastin and collagen? If it doesn't reach the dermis, would it still be able to act as a cofactor in the formation (cross-linking) of collagen and elastin? Would having excess vitamin C present actually affect how much collagen and elastin is being made? Chemical reactions in the body are tightly regulated so it is highly unlikely that adding excess cofactor will have any impact on the amount of collagen being made in the dermis; the amount of cofactor present is not the 'rate-limiting step' in an enzymatic reaction, meaning it is not what controls whether or not a reaction happens.

The bottom line: It has never been shown in normal healthy individuals that taking in more vitamins than required – either orally or topically – has a positive benefit on health.

OTHER BIG SKINCARE CLAIMS FOR VITAMIN C

Vitamin C is often touted as a treatment for pigmentation, but there is no established explanation of how it would work and it seems to be a completely made-up concept by Big Skincare. If you have ever tried to use a vitamin C product to 'brighten' your skin (which is code for 'decrease pigmentation' – kind of like 'getting toned' is code for 'losing body fat' in the fitness industry), you have almost certainly been left disappointed.

And what about photodamage reversal? We know that most skin ageing is due to the sun (photoageing) and the signs of this include fine and deep wrinkles, enlarged pores, brown spots, rough skin texture and dilated capillaries (telangiectasia). How vitamin C would stimulate photodamage reversal is not clear.

The fundamental question is: should you be using a vitamin C product on your skin daily to perhaps protect your skin from oxidative stress or help reverse photodamage, or even increase the amount of collagen and elastin in your dermis? In my opinion, no.

The most important issue for the efficacy of topical application of vitamin C is your blood level of vitamin C; **if you have plenty of vitamin C in your blood, topical application does not increase skin vitamin C content**. The same applies to taking it orally; dietary supplementation of vitamin C only elevates skin vitamin C in people who are deficient.[8]

The bottom line: Using vitamin C topically is almost certainly not necessary for healthy skin (if you are not vitamin C deficient). But it is probably not harmful either.

10

Acids

A cids have been used in skincare for centuries; it is claimed that Cleopatra bathed in sour milk because it softened her skin.[1] But what are acids and can they benefit your skin?

ALPHA-HYDROXY ACIDS

Alpha-hydroxy acids include glycolic, citric, malic and lactic acid. Though often used in peels, here we are going to focus on these acids in cosmetic skincare products.

Glycolic acid

Glycolic acid is the most used alpha-hydroxy acid in skincare. It is primarily used in the treatment of photoaged or photo-damaged skin. A double-blind, randomised clinical trial of the daily use of a 5 per cent glycolic acid formulation applied to the face and neck for a period of three months showed that it provided a mild improvement in general skin texture and dis-colouration.[2] Another double-blind, placebo-controlled study looked to see if 10 per cent glycolic acid applied to the forearm twice daily had any effect on photodamage. Unfortunately, it was found to have no effect at all – the researchers said that it 'appeared almost inactive'.[3]

When used in cosmetic skincare, glycolic acid is usually found in a strength of 2–5 per cent. It is believed to 'work' by reducing the stickiness or 'glue' between the corneocytes of the stratum corneum and stimulate them to flake off. It doesn't seem to do anything to the skin aside from this – it literally just causes injury to the stratum corneum and stimulates exfoliation, especially when used at high concentrations.[4]

What my patients often worry about when using acids is whether they cause issues with how the skin barrier functions, especially if the skin stings after applying them. A study to answer this exact question was devised and involved the twice-daily application of a 4 per cent glycolic acid cream to the forearms of subjects. Biopsies were taken after three weeks of treatment and revealed a more compact stratum corneum, but that transepidermal water loss values did not change. This is great news because it indicates that the barrier function is not compromised by this type of treatment.[5]

So, what is glycolic acid useful for? When used regularly at low concentrations, glycolic acid may possibly enhance the appearance of skin without compromising its function, so this is an ingredient you can look out for in cosmetic skincare products if you want to smooth or 'brighten' your complexion. I often compound glycolic acid 2–4 per cent with hydroquinone in the treatment of solar-induced pigmentation and melasma, to be used in the morning, with a tretinoin-based treatment at night (see Chapter 7). Twice-daily dosing of hydroquinone (see Chapter 8) is important in the initial clearance of pigmentation, and glycolic acid probably enhances the effectiveness of the treatment, without leading to skin dryness or irritation.

SKINTELLIGENT FACT:

What is compounded skincare?

Medicine compounding is the art and science of combining drugs or medicines together into one tablet or

---

cream. You will have come across compounded medicines before – co-codamol (codeine and paracetamol), Augmentin (amoxicillin and clavulanic acid), most cold and cough remedies . . . the list goes on.

Compounding skincare is not a new idea. By combining two creams into one, patients are more compliant with treatment and the two medicines work synergistically so the product is more effective. Epiduo gel (for acne), Fucibet (for infected eczema) and Daktacort (for inflamed fungal infections) are just a few examples of commercially available compounded creams.

True compounding is bespoke and personalised; the doctor decides what medicines are suited for the patient and prescribes the best treatment in the most appropriate concentrations to deal with that specific problem. This requires the doctor to understand the medicines, how they interact and how they 'work' on the skin. And that is an entire skill set on its own!

These creams are 'freshly made', not batch processed, and each patient's treatment is crafted individually. The products have a finite shelf life because they have minimal preservatives added – it's just the medicine and the vehicle. The key to compounding is flexibility; a true compounding lab is capable of making pretty much any combination of strengths the prescriber wants to use (within limits of stability and safety – not all drugs are stable together).

SALICYLIC ACID

Salicylic acid (SA) is a beta-hydroxy acid and is known to have comedone-clearing (comedolytic) as well as antibacterial properties, so it is generally used in the treatment of acne. It is available in different types of cosmetic skincare products from creams to cleansers in up to a 2 per cent strength, but on prescription it can be formulated from 5 to 10 per cent. When seven conventional acne medications were tested to see if they could clear comedones in the skin of acne patients, only two were found to be effective: SA and tretinoin (though tretinoin was more effective than SA – see Chapter 7 for more on tretinoin).[6] It therefore has a role to play in the treatment of mild acne. I often compound 5 per cent SA with 1 per cent clindamycin for my patients with mild to moderate acne in whom other treatments may not be tolerated, and it can be very effective.

Two per cent SA is useful in shampoos and scalp applications to reduce scale in the treatment of dandruff. Using the shampoo twice weekly for five weeks showed a significant decrease in dandruff in all subjects.[7] Topical scalp applications made with 2 per cent SA and a mild steroid are available on prescription and most compounding labs can also make shampoos containing SA, which I regularly prescribe for my patients with dandruff.

AZELAIC ACID

Azelaic acid has become a very trendy ingredient and can be found in a number of cosmetic skincare products in concentrations from 4 to 10 per cent. It is meant to have both antibacterial and anti-inflammatory properties and is purported to be useful in treating everything from acne to melasma.

Though it is a licensed treatment for rosacea when there are papules/pustules present, in strengths of 15 and 20 per cent, it is one of my least prescribed treatments for two reasons: firstly, because we have much better, more effective and targeted treatments for rosacea (see page 206), acne vulgaris (see page 168) and melasma (see page 222) and I would always go for those in the first instance. Secondly, I find that it is extremely irritating to skin.

The only time I use azelaic acid is when treating skin conditions in pregnancy. It can be used for very mild acne vulgaris and can be useful for inflammatory or papulopustular acne, though it's not great for comedonal acne.[8]

Azelaic acid is often prescribed to treat melasma. Though some of the published literature does support its efficacy for melasma, in clinical practice I have not found it to be effective at all. Much better, more efficient and long-lasting clearance of melasma is achieved with compounded creams of tretinoin and hydroquinone (see Chapters 7 and 8).

The bottom line: Though azelaic acid may be helpful for some patients, it is not a great treatment for any one specific thing.

HYALURONIC ACID

The main property of hyaluronic acid (HA) that makes it popular in skincare and aesthetic medicine is its ability to bind a large number of water molecules, thus improving tissue hydration, and to withstand mechanical damage. HA is fully resorbable (meaning over time it becomes absorbed by the body) and biocompatible (meaning the body does not see it as a foreign object and generate an immune response to it).[9]

The average human body weighs 70kg and contains 15g of HA, with the greatest amount being found in the skin. Cosmetic topically applied skincare products containing HA are ubiquitous and widely available; however, so far there have been no randomised controlled studies confirming a positive, long-term smoothing effect on skin or wrinkles from the topical application of HA. In cosmetic preparations, formulations made of HA seemingly 'work' by forming a protective layer over the surface of the skin, making the skin appear softer and feel smoother to the touch – but only temporarily.[10]

You just have to read some of the nonsense skincare companies write on their websites about how their HA product is the most 'advanced' product on the market providing hydration to all the layers of the skin to quickly realise that all this is marketing gibberish and pseudoscience.

There is only one clinical study examining the penetration of HA creams in the epidermis – surprising considering how HA is basically a selling point of virtually every skincare product on the market. Though not a great study due to it being unblinded and uncontrolled with a very small sample size, it showed both high and low molecular weight HA in a cream base did not penetrate the stratum corneum.[11]

> **The bottom line**: Though probably not harmful, HA is another skincare ingredient that is heavily marketed by Big Skincare, but fairly useless when applied to the surface of the skin. Injecting it into the skin is a different matter entirely, though, and is covered on page 264.

11

Other Common Cosmetic Ingredients

As we've seen in the previous four chapters, there are only a handful of ingredients in skincare that actually do anything useful to skin and have a solid scientific evidence base backing them up. On the other hand, there are countless ingredients that fall under the category of 'Totally Useless Things Big Skincare Has Invented to Sell Products'. I feel like every day there is a new product popping up on the market with 'skin-rejuvenating' ingredients derived from sheep placenta, broccoli stem cells or chickpea flour (don't get me started on gold-leaf-infused moisturisers!). And the more complicated or exotic the ingredient sounds, the higher the corresponding price tag. I have chosen three of the newer, more well-known ingredients on the market to critically appraise in this chapter.

COPPER PEPTIDES

Copper peptides are a very trendy skincare ingredient now. Copper is indeed also a cofactor for enzymes, like vitamin C, specifically in the cross-linking of collagen and elastin in the dermis. However, as we've seen, you can't 'speed up' an enzymatic reaction by adding more of a cofactor (see page 141) and, unless you have too little copper hanging out in your dermis, adding more of it does absolutely nothing. This is like having all your building materials for a new house arrive on the same day and expecting the construction to finish earlier. The amount of copper in the skin is not the 'rate-limiting step' in the cross-linking of collagen and elastin – it's not what controls whether or not a reaction happens – so copper peptides applied topically have no function ... another skincare scam. They certainly don't penetrate the dermis where they are meant to work as cofactors either.[1]

The bottom line: This is a great example of another pointless skincare product with a big marketing budget behind it.

BAKUCHIOL

Bakuchiol is an ingredient that is claimed to be a gentler version of retinoic acid. Bakuchiol is derived from the seeds and leaves of the plant *psoralea corylifolia*. It is claimed that it is a 'functional analogue of retinol' because it apparently has a similar effect on cells as that which vitamin A has when added to skin cells in a test tube.[2]

This is an example of how Big Skincare takes an unsubstantiated claim for an ingredient, spins the 'research' to make it sound like 'a new skincare hero', creates products and marketing buzz and ends up making millions of pounds selling, basically, just another moisturiser.

Aside from the fact that cosmetic skincare products made with vitamin A derivatives have no high-quality evidence to back up any of their skincare claims (see page 125), is there any evidence to support that bakuchiol has an impact on skin at all? The answer? No.[3] Despite its presence in an array of cosmetic skincare products, there have been only two studies performed looking at bakuchiol 0.5 per cent cream and its effects on the signs of skin ageing.

The first one had 17 females apply bakuchiol 0.5 per cent cream as a finished skincare product twice daily for 12 weeks. There are many issues with this 'trial', but the major problem is that there was no vehicle control. You *must* have a vehicle control in an efficacy study of anything in order to show that your active ingredient is more effective than just the cream vehicle – moisturising alone every day with *any* moisturiser improves skin roughness, the appearance of fine lines, the smoothness of skin, and so on. Without a vehicle control, the 'results' are completely meaningless. Therefore, though this study showed that the signs of skin ageing improved with the use of the bakuchiol cream after 12 weeks, they would probably have had the same results if they had used plain old Vaseline twice daily for 12 weeks.[4]

The other study compared bakuchiol 0.5 per cent cream to retinol 0.5 per cent cream over 12 weeks in 44 patients.[5] This study was published in the *British Journal of Dermatology*, which is a reputable journal, and it has many positive aspects to its design, but there are again some major issues with how this study was performed and also how the results were analysed, which makes the results suggested by the authors meaningless.

These are what I call 'marketing' studies – they are performed purely to be used as part of the marketing and sale of a product, not to provide any real, informative, scientific data.

Is bakuchiol the new 'skincare hero'? Not based on these publications. It is concerning to see doctors and dermatologists promoting the use of this ingredient when the evidence base for it just doesn't exist. In my opinion, that is poor practice. We shouldn't be helping Big Skincare propagate grossly unsubstantiated claims.[6]

The bottom line: Don't bother with bakuchiol – it has even less 'evidence' for its 'effectiveness' than over-the-counter cosmetic vitamin A derivative products.

NIACINAMIDE

Niacinamide (also known as nicotinamide) is the biologically 'active' form of vitamin B3 (niacin). As a topical, it is claimed to be beneficial for virtually everything – from clearing pigmentation and protecting against UV radiation to being an anti-inflammatory useful for the treatment of rosacea (see page 201) and acne vulgaris (see page 163).

Considering how much effort and money has gone into marketing this topical ingredient, you can be forgiven for thinking that you must use it. But do you really need to? What does the research say?

Not very much, unfortunately. All the 'positive' studies published in the last 15 years showing how effective niacinamide is either have major methodological or statistical analysis flaws or are industry-sponsored or both. Any study not sponsored by industry shows equivocal or negative findings.[7]

A review article looking at the role of nicotinamide in the treatment of acne concluded that 'our review suggests that topical and oral nicotinamide has an unclear effect on acne vulgaris due to the limited nature of available literature'.[8] Another study compared a moisturiser containing niacinamide to pure white petrolatum (Vaseline) and claimed that the niacinamide-laced product reduced transepidermal water loss (TEWL) more than pure petrolatum. As we saw in Chapter 4, Vaseline reduces TEWL by almost 100 per cent, so this finding is extremely hard to believe![9]

The bottom line: You don't need to spend extra cash on a fancy moisturiser that has niacinamide in it or a niacinamide serum to help you get 'better' skin. But if you like the products, they are totally fine to use and not harmful. Just don't expect them to do magic.

WHY YOU SHOULD NEVER BUY COSMETIC SKINCARE PRODUCTS AT YOUR DERMATOLOGIST'S OFFICE

I don't sell skincare products or devices in my clinic. I might do one day, but it will involve lots of mental gymnastics for me to be able to justify it. And before I start to delve into this highly controversial topic, I will say that I am not a saint or a perfect person, but I do work very hard to be the most ethical doctor I can be, and I take that very seriously.

The American Academy of Dermatology has a very clear position statement on this, and the overriding theme is that in-office sale of cosmetic skincare products is ethical *only* when done in a way that is clearly in the patient's best interests.[10] They very clearly state it is unethical to sell cosmetic skincare at the office:

- when the dermatologist has put their own financial interests above the welfare of their patients
- when representing products as being a 'special formulation' not elsewhere available, when this is not the case
- when selling health-related products whose claims of benefit lack validity (which is basically all cosmetic skincare – hello, LED masks!)
- when charging patients an excessive mark-up rate (which is pretty much guaranteed to happen)

The bottom line: Doctors are not profit-maximising entities (or they shouldn't be); unlike normal retail business, doctors exist principally to promote patient health, not maximise profit.

It is important that you, the patient, do not get coerced into buying overpriced, over-hyped cosmetic skincare when you see your dermatologist, believing that products sold at the clinic are in some way better than what you would buy at your local supermarket. And don't feel bad about saying no; you have already paid a fair amount to see the doctor, you don't need to shell out even more for useless cosmetic products that you can also buy for a few quid down the road.

And doctors – if you sell cosmetic products in your clinic, take a moment to think about the ethics of what you are doing and why you became a doctor in the first place: was it to promote patient health or to maximise personal profit?

SKINTELLIGENT TIP:

How to build a skincare routine

Use a cleanser you like that doesn't leave your skin feeling super tight or dry afterwards (I like oil cleansers), and use an SPF in a vehicle you like during the day and use a moisturiser that is as greasy-feeling as you can stand at night.

And don't spend loads of money on any of these products! And that's it.

If you have a skin condition (like acne, rosacea, eczema, pigmentation, melasma, etc) then get a targeted treatment from a doctor.

If you like using and buying skincare and your skin is normal, then go ahead and add in whatever serums/toners/magic potions that you want to, but keep in mind these products are totally unnecessary to keep your skin healthy.

But please do ditch the eye cream, the toner, the gene-modifying serum and the grainy exfoliator. Keep it simple.

PART 4

How to Treat the Most Common Facial Skin Diseases

Skin disease can have a devastating effect on a person's physical and psychological well-being ... from schooling, relationships, self-esteem and career choices to social, sexual and leisure activities.

All Party Parliamentary Group on Skin[1]

The many annoying problems that can affect your skin can drive you to distraction but not to the doctor. Thanks partially to the incessant marketing power of Big Skincare, you may believe that skin problems are simple to correct with a 'well-designed skincare routine' or perhaps a change in your diet. One misguided (and misguiding) 'skinfluencer' even goes so far as to state that 'skin health is a skill you can learn and practice'. If only it were that simple, right?

I see over 6,000 patients a year. My family and close friends (and some of my patients and colleagues) would call me a 'workaholic', but I don't see that as a negative thing. There is nothing more important to me in life than being the best dermatologist I can be. Yes, that might sound a bit lame and yes there is more to life than work (really?!), but this isn't work to me – it's a mission; and my mission is trying to help as many people as possible live their daily lives happy in their own skin.

In this part of the book, we are going to explore in detail the most common facial skin problems and how to treat them. I want to help you stop wasting your time, money and – perhaps most importantly – your hope for better skin on pseudo-science nonsense and marketing hype. I am going to be basing my recommendations for treatments both on what the science and the published evidence say works, and also on my clinical experience.

The two most important parts of treating any skin disease are, first, getting the diagnosis right and, second, making sure you (the patient) understands the treatment plan and helping you stick with it to optimise your results (I call this 'patient compliance'). Both of these things are a dermatologist's responsibility to get right. Your dermatologist is your coach and your cheerleader.

Getting the diagnosis right takes a combination of the doctor's experience, training and visual literacy as well as their ability to examine your skin properly and take an appropriate and thorough history. Getting you to use your treatment requires making sure you understand your diagnosis and the treatment, how it is meant to work, how quickly it should work, what any possible side effects may be, how often to use it, how much to use and what to do if you get side effects. I am a little obsessive about treatment compliance because I know that is the only way my patient will get better – by following the plan!

SKINTELLIGENT FACT:

The cosmetic skincare industry trivialises skin disease – and this can affect your mental health

One of the many issues I have with the cosmetic skincare industry (and people who promote cosmetic skincare) is the trivialising of skin disease. The very idea that a skin disease or skin problem can be solved by a sheet mask or a three-step skincare 'routine' is completely absurd and a blatant lie, but it also downplays the seriousness of the problem: 'Your acne scars are no big deal! Look how easy it is to fix!' For a desperate patient who is devastated by their acne scars, for example, the promise of 'visibly fading scars' in five days sets up an expectation that will absolutely not be met. And if you have ever been massively disappointed by something or someone, you know how horrible that can feel.

Patients with facial skin disease are already vulnerable. Dermatologists performed a study to investigate the mental health of patients with facial skin diseases like acne vulgaris, rosacea, perioral dermatitis and folliculitis.[2] Over 1,000 patients were surveyed and the results were worse than expected: 37.6 per cent of the facial skin disease patients reported having anxiety versus 14.9 per cent of controls; 21.7 per cent reported depression (6.8 per cent in controls); and 9.8 per cent had suicidal ideation (3.2 per cent in controls). Acne patients had the highest levels of anxiety and depression. Most worrying, the patients with the most anxiety and suicidal thoughts were also on average younger than those without.

12

Acne Vulgaris

A cne is a very complex skin disease, and it is also the most common (the word 'vulgaris' is Latin for 'common'), affecting 99 per cent of the population globally at some point. For the sake of simplicity, I am going to refer to acne vulgaris as just 'acne' and to acne spots as 'lesions'.

Virtually every human being on the planet at one point in their life experiences acne (spots, pimples, zits). Acne is a genuine medical, pathologic process but unfortunately most people go to their local department store or chemist for treatment because it is viewed as a 'cosmetic' problem, rather than seeking definitive treatment from an experienced doctor. For the affected person who may also be emotionally vulnerable, one or two red spots and some comedones can be devastating.

SKINTELLIGENT TIP:

There is no such thing as 'mild' acne

Acne is acne and if it bothers you then it should be treated effectively. It's the same for any skin condition: if it affects your quality of life in any way, then it is not a 'small' problem – it's a major problem. When I

---

treat skin conditions I always aim for total clearance, to get my patients' skin back to normal as quickly as possible. Luckily, in the majority of cases, that goal is achievable.

If you are struggling with a skin condition, no matter how 'minor' others may think it is or how often you are told it is a 'normal' part of being a teenager (in the case of acne), this is about your body and how you feel. It doesn't matter what anyone else thinks.

There are four disease-causing (pathogenic) factors involved in the formation of acne lesions:

Follicular hyperkeratinisation

This occurs when there are too many overly sticky skin cells sitting in the hair follicles. How this happens (why the cells are too sticky and don't shed out of the hair follicle like they should) is still up for debate.

Hormonal stimulation of sebaceous glands

Androgen hormones are the sex hormones that people think of as 'male' hormones, and they include testosterone and the more potent dihydrotestosterone. Though high levels of androgens are seen in men, they are also present in women, albeit in much lower concentrations. Androgens are the hormonal drive to developing acne in both men and women, by causing the oil glands attached to the hair follicle to get larger and produce more oil. Generally, androgen blood levels are normal in people with acne; the sebaceous glands appear to be hypersensitive to androgens.[1]

Proliferation of acne bacteria

The increased oil production is a feeding ground for acne bacteria, which causes the bacteria to increase in numbers. If you have acne, you have probably heard of *Propionibacterium acnes* or *P. acnes* – the bacteria that lives in pores and on the skin and is the culprit bacteria in the formation of acne. But have you heard of *Cutibacterium acnes*? This is the 'new' name for *P. acnes*. Same bacteria, new name, as of 2016. Why? Acne is one of the most researched skin diseases and scientists are constantly learning new things about how and why it happens. The version of *P. acnes* that lives on the skin has been found to be genetically different from *P. acnes* that live elsewhere on the body, so scientists created a whole new category of bacteria called *Cutibacterium* to specifically refer to the *P. acnes* group that lives on the skin.[2]

Inflammation

This occurs in response to the increased amount of acne bacteria on the skin.[3]

The image below shows the four stages of the formation of an acne lesion, from early comedone to a pustule (a bump with pus in it that you can see), nodule or cyst. You can see that the build-up of pressure in the follicle leads to the follicle rupturing. The result of this process is a pimple.

The hallmark of acne is that the lesions are polymorphic – meaning that, at any one time, if you have acne, you have lesions at different stages of development. There are two main types of acne lesions: inflammatory and non-inflammatory. Inflammatory lesions are red, painful, hot and often have pus in them (called pustules) and they can also be deep, 'under the skin' cystic nodules. Non-inflammatory lesions are comedones (open and closed) and are not red. Some comedones will turn into inflammatory lesions, some will go away on their own and some

THE FOUR STAGES OF THE FORMATION OF AN ACNE LESION

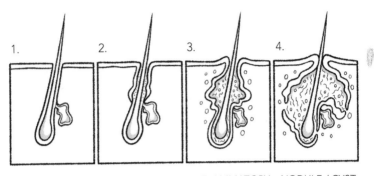

EARLY COMEDONE	LATER COMEDONE	INFLAMMATORY PAPULE	NODULE / CYST

will just stay as they are. Extracting comedones can potentially bring on inflammatory acne because you are disrupting the hair follicle lining and the trapped cells, which can then cause the hair follicle to rupture and lead to an inflammatory lesion.

It takes about 13 days for an active inflammatory lesion to go away – there is not a lot you can do to speed up its resolution except to leave it alone. That means *no picking*! There is actually a medical diagnosis for people who pick at their acne – it's called acne excoriée. It's something I diagnose a lot more often than I want to! You know without me telling you that picking just prolongs the misery of each and every single spot you get and increases the chances of it leaving a mark or even a permanent scar.[4]

Acne tends to only occur in areas of high sebaceous gland concentration in association with vellus hair follicles (the finer, lighter hairs that cover most of your face and body), as opposed to terminal hair follicles (the darker, thicker ones). Generally, people don't get acne on their scalps even though the scalp has the greatest density of sebaceous glands anywhere on the body. The reason is that on your scalp, the wide, fat terminal hairs fill up the entire hair follicle canals and do not allow the accumulation of oil and keratin debris to build up into a comedone.

On the face, however, we mainly have vellus hairs that are

very thin and fine and do not fully obstruct the hair follicle canal, therefore allowing for the accumulation of keratin and oil to form a comedone. Patients often ask me why they only get acne on their forehead or their cheeks. One explanation for this is because that is where you have lots of sebaceous glands and vellus hairs.

SKINTELLIGENT TIP:

There are only two reasons to 'pop' a pimple

1. To relieve pain. Often, cystic acne lesions can be extremely painful. Ideally, you would not try to 'pop' it or extract the cyst contents, but sometimes the pain is so bad it is the only way to feel better - but there is no good technique for this (the one explained in the point below isn't great for cysts because there is no whitehead specifically). The risk of bad scarring is high, which is why this is generally a bad idea. If you have a painful, sore, inflamed spot it's best to get it injected by a dermatologist with a little bit of intralesional steroid. It will go down dramatically within a few hours when done correctly. Definitely see a consultant dermatologist if you want to go down this route. Otherwise, just leave it alone - it will get better!
2. For cosmetic reasons. Having a whitehead filled with pus on your face is just not very pretty to look at. If you want to get rid of the pus, use a very fine sterile needle and, with clean hands, very gently stick the needle straight into the top of the spot.

This should not hurt. Then use cotton buds to gently press on either side to extract the contents. Try not to just squeeze them with your fingers because this damages the surrounding skin and will just make the whole thing a big mess.

Your best bet, of course, is to just leave it alone. Most spots resolve after a few days (13, on average), but the big painful 'under the skin' cysts can last for a few weeks.

TREATMENTS

Topicals

Topical treatments for acne include benzoyl peroxide, antibiotics (clindamycin and erythromycin), combinations of benzoyl peroxide and antibiotics, retinoids (see Chapter 7) and acids like salicylic and azelaic acid (see Chapter 10). Combination therapies that are commercially available are usually more effective than single agents. Generally, topicals alone can be helpful for mild acne and as maintenance treatment once clearance has been achieved using more potent treatments.

Topical treatments for acne should be used on the entire face (so even on areas where you don't have spots) and not as a spot treatment. We know from biopsy studies that the skin around the active acne spots (perilesional skin) in acne patients exhibits evidence of subclinical inflammation, meaning you can't see the redness or irritation at the skin surface. In other words, the problems that cause individual acne lesions affect the entire skin of an acne patient, not just that one small area where the lesion is present. Topical acne treatments work in various ways to reduce inflammation, reduce sebum secretion and 'unstick' the cells that are clogging the hair follicles.

It can be argued that once an acne lesion has developed and is an active, inflamed, red lesion, the 'ship has sailed' in terms of the efficacy of acne treatments to improve the situation. In fact, using topical acne medications on fully inflamed lesions potentially further irritates already irritated skin, causing issues with wound healing, and can lead to worse scarring once the inflammation has gone down. This, in turn, might be the reason why acne appears to 'get worse' at the beginning of acne treatment with a topical retinoid.

We know that there are a number of reasons why topical retinoids cause skin irritation, which is called 'retinoid dermatitis' (see page 128). Overwhelming the skin cells' retinoic acid receptors at the start of treatment acutely affects the functioning and structure of the epidermis. We also know that an already impaired barrier function (also known as 'skin barrier dysfunction') is probably one of the key underlying problems seen in acne. Therefore, it might not be unreasonable to say that the reason acne lesions might flare at the start of retinoid treatment is due to the irritation of pre-existing lesions by the topical treatment. Once a full-blown inflammatory cascade is in motion, not much can be done to dampen that down aside from giving it time to settle on its own.

Additionally, when patients seek professional medical advice for their skin condition, they are usually quite a bit more motivated to 'look after themselves' in order to get the most from their treatment. This, in turn, can lead patients to begin utilising several new treatments and products. As mentioned, skin barrier dysfunction is now thought of as a key factor in causing acne in the first place and using lots of various 'lotions and potions' on skin at the same time as prescription treatment may lead to a temporary flare-up of acne lesions.

Finally, acne is a cyclical, relapsing and remitting skin condition that is hormonally controlled. When starting a new treatment, patients are hyper-aware of any changes and are also looking for an overnight improvement – both of which can predispose them to thinking they are having an acne 'flare' due to treatment, which in fact is only 'flaring' due to its cyclical nature or because the patient is just paying more attention.

I generally say that you need to give topical acne treatments at least 12 weeks of consistent use before saying they don't work. And by consistent use I mean nightly or alternate nights without adding in various other 'treatments' at the same time (facials, lasers, microdermabrasion, topical acid preparations, and so on).

SKINTELLIGENT TIP:

How to prevent the 'retinoid purge'

The dreaded 'retinoid purge' refers to a usually brief episode of a flare-up of acne pustules at the start of using a topical retinoid. I don't see this in my patients very often, but it is something widely discussed in blogs and on social media.

The first thing is knowing why this happens: the new spots are probably due to how the retinoid works – it breaks down the stuck-together skin cells of the comedones quickly, which results in the formation of a spot. This is actually a sign that the retinoid is getting into the hair follicle unit and doing what it needs to do.[5] But it is disheartening and upsetting for patients at the start of treatment.

So, what can you do to prevent this from happening? I suggest the following tactics (and this is potentially why many of my patients don't experience this problem):

- Start with a low-strength tretinoin or adapalene (see Chapter 7) and start using it on alternate

---

days only for a few weeks and slowly increase to using it nightly.

- I almost always prescribe oral antibiotics at the same time as commencing a topical retinoid for acne, which can potentially help reduce the risk of the 'purge' but also help clear the acne more quickly.
- If you have a choice between adapalene or tretinoin, go for adapalene in the first instance if you are concerned about a purge. Though all retinoids can lead to a purge, there is some evidence to suggest that adapalene can also work to reduce some inflammation in the skin, which might make it less likely than tretinoin to cause a purge at the start of treatment.[6]

The important thing to remember is to stick with your treatment despite the flare-up: know that this can potentially happen to you and be mentally prepared for it. If it gets really out-of-hand, speak to your doctor about more ways to minimise it.

Adapalene or tretinoin?

Both adapalene and tretinoin are retinoic acid – so the active vitamin A derivative (see Chapter 7). But you might be wondering how they are different and, if you are trying to manage your acne, which one you should go for. The difference between the two is based on which retinoic acid receptors the medicine acts on.

Adapalene binds mainly to the RAR beta and gamma receptors, while tretinoin binds all RAR subtypes (though also preferentially to gamma). The gamma receptor is the one that regulates how the skin cells in the hair follicle function so that's why adapalene was specifically created for acne.

We have good clinical trial evidence to show that adapalene does indeed improve acne.[7] But is it just as good as or better than tretinoin for acne? That's a great question, but unfortunately there is no answer yet. It is also claimed that adapalene is less irritating than tretinoin, but the clinical trial evidence is not 100 per cent sure about that one either.

So, what do you do? If you have acne, I suggest that most people start with adapalene because it is commercially available on prescription in the UK combined in one product with benzoyl peroxide (and easily available from your NHS GP), and benzoyl peroxide is the most powerful topical treatment for acne. (Benzoyl peroxide cannot be combined in one cream with tretinoin because of stability issues.) However, if that is not available to you and tretinoin is, then go for tretinoin because we know it does the job for acne too. You would then use a separate benzoyl peroxide product on its own in the morning, if necessary. There is nothing yet to suggest one is better than the other for acne.[8]

Light therapies

Cochrane reviews of medical topics provide high-quality, independent evidence to inform healthcare decision-making. In 2017, a Cochrane review was published investigating light therapies for acne – specifically the safety and effectiveness of things like blue- and red-light therapy.[9] When blue light was compared to the use of 5 per cent benzoyl peroxide, no significant difference in outcome was found. The conclusion of the review was that no light therapy could be recommended for the treatment of acne. Considering how expensive light treatment is compared to standard prescription topical treatment, based on the available evidence **I would not recommend my acne patients spend time and money on light treatments**. Don't be tempted to buy one of those light masks you see advertised for sale all over the internet right now either – it is a total marketing gimmick and won't help your acne.

Oral antibiotics

Oral antibiotics have been a fundamental part of acne treatment for decades. This is very controversial and, potentially, we should not be using them anymore as they are generally not incredibly effective for anything but mild acne or patients who have never had any type of prescribed acne treatment before. It's usually the first thing patients get when they go to their doctor with acne.

Cutibacterium acnes bacterium lives on the skin and in the pores and hair follicles, and it survives by eating fatty acids in the sebum (oil) that is produced by the sebaceous glands in your hair follicles. When there is increased oil production in the skin, *C. acnes* bacteria grow and multiply. How *C. acnes* contributes to acne is fairly complex: the bacteria secrete lots of proteins, including digestive enzymes, which can work to 'eat away' at the walls of hair follicles. The mess of cell debris this leaves behind can then trigger an inflammatory response in the body that leads to the signs and symptoms of acne.

This damage to the hair follicle and the associated inflammation caused by *C. acnes* makes the skin more easily infected by other bacteria. There is some new research showing that normal, healthy skin pores are only colonised by *C. acnes*, while in acne the pores are also colonised by staphylococcus species.[10] How relevant this is to the development of acne is not known, but it is important to note that when we use antibiotics to treat acne, we are doing so to reduce the *C. acnes* load and thus the accompanying inflammation and damage produced by it in the hair follicle, not necessarily to get rid of the *C. acnes* itself. The antibiotics have an anti-inflammatory effect rather than a purely antibacterial effect on acne.

C. acnes is sensitive to a huge range of antibiotics and

antibacterial agents. Tetracyclines like lymecycline are the ones commonly prescribed. Acne treatment guidelines recommend starting treatment with oral antibiotics for inflammatory acne, but only when combined with a topical agent – and that topical agent should have benzyl peroxide in it. My favoured starting regime is oral lymecycline and a topical combination treatment of adapalene 0.1 per cent and benzoyl peroxide 2.5 per cent. If at three months, acne has improved more than 50 per cent, the antibiotic can be continued for a further three months. If there has been no or minimal improvement, it should be stopped, and no new antibiotic started. A new, different treatment should be considered.

SKINTELLIGENT FACT:

The truth about antibiotic resistance

My patients often ask me whether it is safe to take antibiotics for many months, and this is also a popular topic on social media. The antibiotic resistance issue is controversial and confusing. At an individual patient level, it does not mean very much, but it does on a population level. When we talk about antibiotic resistance, it is not in reference to the antibiotic no longer working for you as an individual patient; it's about it not working if someone gets very ill from an infection by a bacterium that is resistant to the antibiotics we use for acne and there are no other suitable treatments. This can potentially mean that a 'superbug' can develop in the future for which we will have no suitable treatment. For the individual, however, it is safe to take antibiotics specifically made for acne for a number of months.

Hormonal

We know that the contraceptive pill helps with acne by suppressing sebum production in the skin. This effect is facilitated by the oestrogens in the pill lowering the circulating level of testosterone (one of the androgen hormones). A 2012 Cochrane review confirmed that the combined birth control pill (that has both oestrogen and progesterone) is effective in the treatment of both inflammatory and non-inflammatory (comedonal) acne.[11] Importantly, they found no difference in efficacy with regards to acne between the different types of combined contraceptive pill – including special 'acne' ones like Dianette. (Dianette is a type of combined pill that has cyproterone acetate in it – an 'anti-androgen' – and is licensed for the treatment of severe acne.)

If you have been on Dianette, you may have had it stopped by your doctor after one or two years of treatment. That's because it increases the risk of blood clots (venous thromboembolism) – the risk has been found to be 1.5–2 times higher than for some other types of combined pills – so doctors don't like to keep patients on it for a very long time.[12]

The progestogen-only pill (the 'mini' pill) tends to make acne worse though, so if you need contraception and want something to help your acne, try to avoid this type of pill.

Spironolactone is a diuretic that, at higher doses, has an anti-androgen effect. It is an FDA-approved drug for the treatment of acne. The usual dosing starts at 50mg and goes up to 200mg per day, depending on the patient's response. Though there are no randomised placebo-controlled trials of it in adult female acne, there have been observational and retrospective case series that demonstrate its safety and efficacy. In one study of 139 patients treated for 20 weeks at a dose range of 100–200mg per day, 100 per cent of patients had a positive response with a reduction in acne lesions, 50 per cent of whom had an excellent response with significant improvement.[13] If you cannot take the combined pill for whatever reason or just don't want to and have mild to moderate acne, spironolactone may be a good option for you. I often prescribe it as maintenance therapy to my female patients after they attain clearance of their acne with oral isotretinoin (see below).

SKINTELLIGENT FACT:

Stopping the pill and acne

A lot of women come to see me when they need to come off the combined contraceptive pill for whatever reason and they have been on it to control their acne.

There are two main things that can happen from a dermatology perspective when you stop taking the pill: you can get acute hair shedding in the form of telogen effluvium, but this is almost always temporary (6–12 months) and does not result in baldness.

The other problem is the acne flare-up and I refer to this as 'post-contraceptive acne'. It usually starts 3–4 months after stopping the pill. The acne mainly consists of inflammatory papules and pustules (not a lot of blackheads, nodules or cysts), and generally occurs on the lower cheeks and chin. This usually settles down after 6–12 months on its own (without treatment), but it can be more severe in women who had acne as teenagers.

This is, of course, generally super distressing. The best way to deal with it is to use a topical retinoid (if there is no reason not to do so, referred to as a 'contraindication') preferably *before* you stop the pill and then if that is not enough to control it to move on to more intensive treatment, like adding in benzoyl peroxide or oral antibiotics, or even considering oral isotretinoin.

Sometimes spironolactone can help. The main difficulty is that patients who stop the pill generally want to do so because they are planning on trying for a baby. If that is the case, then switching to pregnancy-safe acne treatments like azelaic acid (see page 150) along with super-basic, minimal skincare can be the answer. Always consult your dermatologist for specific advice.

Basic skincare (adjunctive therapy)

As we've seen, filaggrin is a key protein in the structure and function of the stratum corneum (see page 14). Within acne lesions, there is an increase in the amount of filaggrin present in keratinocytes (skin cells) lining the hair follicle wall. In addition, acne bacteria have been shown to increase the filaggrin in cultured keratinocytes. We now know that the normal-looking (unaffected by acne) skin of patients with acne is often inflamed in a similar way to the skin just around the acne lesion itself. Also, research has found that patients with acne have higher sebum secretion but also greater transepidermal water loss with lower stratum corneum hydration than those without acne, which supports the concept that barrier dysfunction has a role to play in acne.[14] Then if we add into the mix a topical treatment like benzoyl peroxide or a retinoid that can temporarily irritate the skin and cause further barrier dysfunction, we are creating a problem. That's where cleansers and moisturisers come in as 'adjunctive' or supportive therapy when we treat acne.

Cleansing

First and foremost – acne is absolutely *not* caused by dirt on the skin. Cleansing to remove dirt to try to combat acne doesn't make sense and can actually irritate the skin and make acne worse. **You cannot 'scrub away' acne lesions, comedones or blackheads – stay away from grainy scrubs or exfoliating washes.**

There is virtually no scientific evidence to support the idea that routinely washing your face twice a day even with a mild cleanser is specifically beneficial if you have acne. In fact, repeated exposure of the skin to water alone may disturb the epidermal barrier function, causing dehydration, irritation, changes to the skin pH and alteration of the normal skin flora.

A pivotal study in 1980 identified skin dryness as an aggravating factor in both the cause and the successful treatment of acne. The researchers compared a programme of topical tretinoin and benzoyl peroxide with water avoidance (so no cleansing) with a programme of oral antibiotic therapy and topical tretinoin and another programme of oral antibiotic therapy with the use of a cleanser. After 16 weeks in all groups, the degree of dryness was directly correlated with lack of improvement, and they concluded that the topical-only programme with water avoidance and no cleansing was the most effective at treating acne.[15]

Though no cleansing is not a bad idea, most patients probably would not go for that, especially if they wear make-up. In addition, gentle cleansing at night removes sunscreen and make-up that can interfere with the absorption of the night-time prescription acne treatments you are using. **Choose a very mild cleanser (like an oil cleanser) and use it once or twice a day at most, but cleansing alone is not the solution to clearing your acne.** Avoid antibacterial cleansers because they do not actually decrease the amount of acne bacteria on the skin and may promote the development of folliculitis (inflammation of the hair follicles, which leads to the development of small pustules that look like acne spots!) if the balance of skin bacteria is unnecessarily shifted.[16] You do not need to use an oil-free cleanser; an oil cleanser is perfectly acceptable. However, if the idea of putting oil on your skin still scares you, there are a lot of options for inexpensive, gentle cleansers for you to choose from. Just go for one that you like to use.

Moisturising

Dry skin can make acne worse, but it can be brought on by the use of anti-acne topical treatments. However, when you have oily, shiny skin with spots, I totally understand that the last thing you want to apply is more oil via a moisturiser. As we've seen, moisturisers work by occluding the skin surface and keeping water in the skin (see pages 70–77). Using an 'oil-free' moisturiser is not necessary; this term is totally inaccurate as there is no legal or regulatory definition of it or even an industry standard of what 'oil-free' actually means.[17] **My preferred moisturiser is (no surprise here!) Vaseline – even for acne patients** (see page 76 for more on this). Start out by using just a very thin layer of it on top of your night-time acne treatment. I promise it won't make you break out!

Oral isotretinoin

Oral isotretinoin (also known under the brand names Roaccutane, Accutane and Oratane) is a retinoid and is the gold-standard treatment for acne. It is by far the most effective treatment available, the one with the most unbiased scientific evidence base for safety and efficacy as well as the one dermatologists have the most experience using and getting virtually 100 per cent acne clearance with (when used correctly and tailored for the specific patient's needs). We also have a very good understanding of how it works.

European guidelines strongly recommend the use of oral isotretinoin in moderate to severe papulopustular (papules and pustules) and nodular (abscesses that feel deep in the skin) acne at a dose of 0.3–0.5mg/kg/day. Isotretinoin can be used in the management of acne that meets one or more of the following criteria:[18]

- severe nodulocystic acne
- severe papulopustular acne

- moderate to severe nodular acne
- minimal response to previous treatments
- prone to significant scarring
- sudden relapse after stopping therapy
- patients with significant psychological distress
- moderate inflammatory acne with resulting physical or psychological scarring[19]

The bottom line: Isotretinoin does the job and does it safely for the most part, so if you have acne that has not cleared with 'standard' treatment, it is an option worth exploring with an experienced consultant or board-certified dermatologist who can help you decide if it is the right treatment for you.

How does isotretinoin work?

There are retinoic acid receptors on the sebocytes (the cells of the oil glands) and isotretinoin activates these receptors, causing the sebocyte to shrink and sometimes disappear completely. Histological studies (when skin samples are examined under a microscope) have shown that isotretinoin causes the large cauliflower-like sebaceous glands abundant in the skin of acne patients to shrink down to small little buds. This also leads to a reduction of acne bacteria on the skin since the bacteria normally feed off the oil to survive. There are multiple positive effects of isotretinoin on the skin of patients with acne and they include:

- reduced size of sebaceous glands
- reduced sebum production of sebaceous glands
- normalisation of follicular keratinisation
- inhibition of the growth of acne bacteria through a change in environment in the hair follicle
- an associated reduction of inflammation

Isotretinoin also alters the composition of the lipids (oil) secreted onto the skin – glycerides are reduced and cholesterol levels increase, among other changes, leading to a reduction in comedones.[20]

SKINTELLIGENT TIP:

How I manage my patients on isotretinoin

The first thing my patients want to know is 'How long will I be taking it?' My answer to that is usually 6-9 months, unless the acne is severe, then closer to a year. The aim of the treatment is that your skin is completely clear of acne - with not a single spot. Therefore, I want my patients to not have a single spot for at least four weeks before we either stop treatment or slowly start to reduce the dose. If they get a spot while the dose is going down, then I know they need to be on it for a little longer. I usually also start a topical retinoid when I start the dose reduction plan and, sometimes, I also start spironolactone for some of my female patients (see page 177). The aim is to get the skin to be completely clear and then to keep it that way in the long run.

The capsules should be taken at night with food and if you miss a day or two you don't then double up on the dose the next day. I generally keep most patients on a low dose, to minimise any side effects like dry lips. To reduce the risk of a bad flare at the start of treatment, if a patient has very severe acne or lots of comedones, I may add in some extra different treatments at the beginning to minimise any flare-ups.

And, yes, you can wear make-up while taking it, but I always recommend absolutely minimal skincare with a very basic cleanser once daily, a greasy ointment moisturiser at night and sunscreen during the day. And that's it. Occasionally, if a patient has melasma or lots of post-inflammatory pigmentation spots from previous acne, I will also start them on a compounded treatment to use at night to help with the pigmentation while the acne is being cleared.

The first thing all patients notice (within a week or two of starting) is a dramatic reduction in oiliness – both of the skin and the scalp. After that, the spots will start to improve, but noticeable improvement normally takes at least 2–3 months of consistent treatment. I know patients with acne are impatient to get clear skin, so I have to make sure they understand the time scale and the importance of not trying to 'speed things up' by using extra 'acne treatments' or getting facials. While on isotretinoin, don't do anything else – just let the treatment work.

And, yes, you can drink alcohol while taking it (though it needs to be in moderation – no more than 14 units a week as per the British Association of Dermatologists and UK government guidance).[21]

Medications to avoid while taking isotretinoin are tetracycline antibiotics, methotrexate and vitamin A supplements. If isotretinoin is taken with tetracyclines, there is a risk of a rise in pressure of the fluid around the brain (known as increased intracranial pressure), so you must stop your tetracycline antibiotics at least four weeks before starting treatment with isotretinoin.

Side effects of isotretinoin

The side effects of isotretinoin can be separated into specific categories. The first and most relevant category is that if isotretinoin is taken by pregnant women, it can cause foetal malformations, premature birth or spontaneous abortion. This is known as 'teratogenicity'. Note that isotretinoin is not a hormonal drug and does not affect a woman's ability to get pregnant or her periods. Because it can cause birth defects, if you are of childbearing age, you must be taking some form of definitive contraception (like the combined contraceptive pill or an intrauterine device as well as using condoms) if you are sexually active. If you are on isotretinoin and would like to get pregnant, you need to stop taking the medication for at least four weeks before trying to conceive.[22]

The second – and most common – category of side effects are short-term 'mucocutaneous' side effects – that's dryness of the skin and mucous membranes, like the lips and inside the mouth, nose and eyelids. Patients on isotretinoin also have a tendency to angular cheilitis (cracks at the corners of the mouth that don't heal because of the candida sitting in the cracks) while on treatment. The isotretinoin reduces the skin's oil secretion and causes the lips to get dry and cracked. The lack of antimicrobial sebum then allows the candida that normally lives in the mouth to infect those cracks and stop them from healing. An altered barrier function as well as 'corneocyte decohesion' – which means the stratum corneum cells are more easily separated and shed off, which also increases TEWL – leads to more skin dryness. In my experience, when the dose is appropriately tailored for the patient, skin dryness is generally very minimal. However, there is a temporary loss of the antioxidant barrier with the decrease in skin surface oil, which leads to increased risk of burning with sunlight exposure. That's why, if you are on isotretinoin, you are at an increased risk of burning if you go out in the sun. Another reason to cover up and wear your sunscreen! These mucocutaneous side effects tend to occur more severely in patients when the drug dose is higher than 0.5mg/kg per day.

Acne can also get a bit worse in the first month of treatment and, very rarely, a temporary increase in hair shedding can occur, known as telogen effluvium. The idea that isotretinoin causes dramatic hair loss is not accurate. Vitamin A, at normal levels, is necessary because it helps the hair follicle and sebaceous gland to function the way it should. However, in the case of vitamin A toxicity, hair loss is inevitable. In clinical trials, when isotretinoin is dosed appropriately (0.5mg/kg per day) for three months of treatment, hair was not affected and no patient experienced alopecia. This supports the fact that isotretinoin does not alter hair growth.[23]

The third category of side effects are 'extracutaneous' side effects – not relating to the skin. These include headaches, muscle or joint aches. Low back pain is one of the very common side effects of isotretinoin. Isotretinoin-induced low back pain is dose-related; the average dose of isotretinoin was significantly higher in patients found to have low back pain in clinical trials than in patients without low back pain.[24] There have been some reports that there is an association between inflammatory bowel disease (colitis) and taking isotretinoin, but we know this is not the case. In an analysis of six research studies, there was no increased risk of developing inflammatory bowel disease in patients exposed to isotretinoin compared with patients not exposed to isotretinoin.[25] Furthermore, there was no increased risk of developing Crohn's disease or ulcerative colitis in patients exposed to isotretinoin compared with those not exposed to the medication.

Blood tests are required prior to commencing treatment and at specific intervals during treatment. An increase in blood cholesterol and triglyceride levels as well as a temporary increase in liver enzyme markers (the proteins your liver makes to, for example, produce bile or help break down the food you eat) can occur. A large meta-analysis found that oral isotretinoin was associated with a temporary increase in blood cholesterol levels, but not high enough to be of any concern.[26] In addition, the proportion of patients with such change in levels was low enough that it was deemed not necessary to check this monthly (as stated in the EU summary of product characteristics). You will need blood tests before starting treatment, after 6–8 weeks of treatment and then every 3 months during treatment.

Though there are some concerns around wound healing while taking isotretinoin, there is no good evidence to suggest that oral isotretinoin causes issues with wound healing post-surgery. However, if you are on treatment and need surgery, it is best to speak to your surgeon about what they would like you to do with regards to your acne treatment.[27]

By far one of the most common questions I get about acne treatment is about the effect of oral isotretinoin on mood. Patients are often scared of taking this medication because of all the bad press it gets about it causing mental health problems like depression and suicide, but where has this idea come from? We've seen that having acne has a substantial psychological impact on most patients with the condition, manifesting mainly as depressive symptoms (see page 161). One study published in 1983 suggested that oral isotretinoin could cause depressive symptoms and, since then, multiple publications have fuelled the controversy on this subject.[28] Those studies that found a positive association between isotretinoin and depression concluded that it occurred in a minority of patients who often had a personal history or family history of depression.[29] However, most studies have *not* found an association between oral isotretinoin and depression but, rather, have found a beneficial effect of reduced depressive symptoms with the treatment.[30] Acne patients on isotretinoin experience fewer depressive symptoms and psychological distress when compared to those treated with oral antibiotics, and studies have shown that depression decreased significantly in patients treated with isotretinoin after completing treatment and this improvement began when treatment began.[31]

There is no evidence to suggest that exposure to isotretinoin actually *causes* adverse psychiatric effects, such as depressive disorder, mood swings and anxiety disorders. It's important to remember that mental health problems often have lots of causes, and are unfortunately very common in teenagers and especially in teenagers with severe acne.

SKINTELLIGENT TIP:

You can get laser hair removal while on isotretinoin

The 2017 American Society for Dermatological Surgery Task Force reported the following: 'there is insufficient evidence to justify delaying treatment with superficial chemical peels and non-ablative lasers, including hair removal lasers and lights, vascular lasers and non-ablative fractional devices for patients currently or recently exposed to isotretinoin'.[32] And, yes electrolysis for hair removal is fine too!

Dosing

Though isotretinoin has been approved for the treatment of acne since 1982, there is still uncertainty about the ideal or optimal dose. Through my clinical experience, I have learnt that for most patients a relatively low dose (0.5mg/kg or less) over a longer period (8–12 months) is better tolerated and more effective at clearing skin and keeping side effects to an absolute minimum than a higher dose (1mg/kg) for a shorter period of time (4–6 months). I also find that the low-dose/long-course method leads to a lower chance of relapse after stopping. I don't use a 'target' cumulative dose, but rather aim for my patients to have no lesions at all for at least four weeks before we start thinking about slowly reducing the dose or stopping it.

My approach is not just based on my own practice, but is also evidence-based (of course!). The question about dosing is really about what is optimal to reduce the risk of relapse after stopping the treatment – and that's what all my patients are most concerned about.

One review found no significant difference in therapeutic result between any of the dosing groups – though there was some evidence to suggest that, in patients with severe acne, a higher dose was better than a lower dose for a fixed amount of time.[33]

When looking at relapse rates, it doesn't seem to matter if the cumulative dose (the total amount of medication taken over the treatment period) is under or over 120mg/kg. The most recent international consensus on isotretinoin dosage makes no specific recommendations on dosing at all; they simply recommend continuing isotretinoin until full clearance of acne is achieved, plus an additional month, independent of cumulative dose.[34]

The bottom line: It doesn't matter if you go low and slow or go high and fast when it comes to isotretinoin dosage. However, for most patients, lower dosages given over a longer period of time will result in similar outcomes and significantly fewer adverse effects – and that's what I recommend for most patients.

ACNE IN TEENAGERS

My message to teenagers with acne is that, first of all, it can be fixed – and it can be fixed relatively quickly (give it 2–3 months to start seeing good clearance). But you almost certainly will not find the cure you are after via a ten-step skincare programme, a set of skincare you buy at a department store, an

LED light mask (don't even get me started!) or, probably, at the hands of a well-meaning facialist or beautician. And please don't take your skincare advice from YouTube and TikTok!

Acne is a skin disease and needs to be treated as such. If the treatment from your GP or healthcare professional isn't helping, consider seeing a consultant or board-certified dermatologist.

A few key things to remember include:

- If you have tried a six-month course of antibiotics and it hasn't worked, then you need something that's not an antibiotic. Even the acne treatment guidelines for doctors do *not* recommend switching 'types' of antibiotics to get a response. If one type failed, move on. There is no data that suggests one antibiotic is better at treating acne than another.
- Antibiotics for acne need to be taken continuously for at least three months to see a response *and* combined with a topical treatment like benzoyl peroxide.
- Antibiotics do *not* cure acne (except in the very few with mild acne) – if they work for you, that's great, but you will almost certainly need to take them for a very long time to keep your acne away (and probably once you stop taking them your acne will come back).
- When it comes to topical treatments for acne, the most effective one is benzoyl peroxide – 2.5 per cent is usually strong enough.
- The only topical treatment that *may* improve comedones is a topical retinoid, but it takes a very long time (we are talking months) of daily use to see an improvement.
- If you are female, consider going on the combined oral contraceptive pill to improve your acne (progestogen-only ones can make acne worse).
- Facials do *not* help acne and there is evidence to suggest that they can actually cause acne 6–8 weeks post-facial in up to a third of people.[35]

- No topical treatment will permanently improve oily skin.
- 'Medicated' acne cleansers are a total waste of time – just use something that is bland and non-irritating (and inexpensive).
- If your skin is feeling tight after cleansing, you have 'over-cleansed' – your skin needs some oil on it!
- If you start getting scarring, you need a more powerful treatment to clear your acne. Acne scarring can be very difficult to fix.
- Don't be scared of oral isotretinoin – speak to a doctor to discuss this treatment and to see if it is right for you. There is a lot of misinformation on social media and the internet about this medicine, so please don't believe everything you read.

ACNE IN ADULT WOMEN

One thing I notice in my clinics, but also through observing people generally, is that adult females get acne a lot more commonly than adult males (in this context, an adult is someone over 25 years old). Over 50 per cent of women in their twenties have acne and almost 30 per cent of women over 40 have acne as well.[36] Female patients account for two thirds of visits made to a dermatologist for acne and one third of all dermatology visits for acne are by women older than 25 years.

Why is that? We know that raised blood levels of androgens (the one we think of as the 'male' hormone, but women have low levels of it too) cause acne in teenage girls. Importantly, physical or psychological stress is known to be a stimulus for your adrenal glands to produce more androgens as well. Is this because adult women are more stressed than adult men? Maybe – but certain adult women may be more sensitive to androgens than men (remember there are also androgen receptors on scalp hair follicles).

It is easy to blame everything on stress, but I do think some women are more sensitive to stress-induced fluctuations of hormones and that may partially account for some women's adult acne problems (and even possibly hair thinning).

'Period' spots

It seems to be common knowledge that the chin and jawline is the place where women get 'hormonal' acne – namely around our periods. But why is that? Isn't all acne due to hormones?

Dr C. Griffiths, a leading UK consultant dermatologist, wrote a very interesting paper exploring this very topic.[37] He describes a 'triangle of hormone sensitivity' on the chin. In this area, an artery known as the mental artery provides a rich blood supply to the overlying skin. Using thermal imaging, Dr Griffiths showed that this coincides with 'hot spots' for blood flow. This increased blood flow means that there is an 'overabundant and continuous supply of androgens to the area'. He does state that there might be an increased density of androgen receptors at this area as well, meaning there are more cells that can respond to the androgen hormone signal specifically in this area.

I always like to know the 'why' and I found this to be a compelling explanation for why we get spots on our chin/jawline around our period. I've found that the best way to manage it is by controlling the hormone fluctuations, and Dr Griffiths also suggests using 'topical oestrogen creams', but also that 'low-dose isotretinoin has proved most valuable'.

This may make you think, 'Oh I should get my hormone levels checked' – you are not alone in thinking this! When they come to see me, over half of my female acne patients bring all their 'hormone blood work' with them to show me that it is all normal! And, of course, I am not surprised. So here is the question: if you have acne, do you need to get your hormone levels checked? As Dr Albert Kligman said, 'Acne is not due to that favourite old dodge "hormone imbalance". It is not, except in very rare cases, an endocrinologic disorder and no money should be wasted on futile laboratory studies . . .'[38]

TRIANGLE OF HORMONE SENSITIVITY AND BLOOD SUPPLY TO CHIN

TRIANGLE OF HORMONE SENSITIVITY

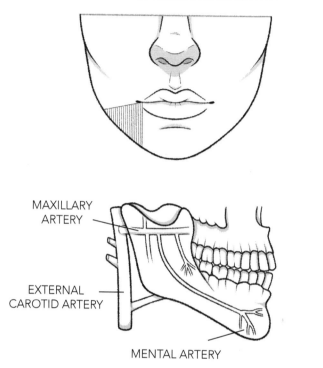

MAXILLARY ARTERY

EXTERNAL CAROTID ARTERY

MENTAL ARTERY

The bottom line: Most women with acne do *not* need to get their hormone levels checked.

We know it is not the level of androgens in the blood that are driving the acne. What is happening is that **the sebaceous glands in acne-prone people are hypersensitive to androgens**; that means that in some people, the same level of androgens will cause their oil glands to enlarge and produce more oil, setting off a cascade of events leading to an acne lesion, but in some people this doesn't happen to the same extent. Therefore, hormone levels in acne patients will invariably always be normal.

With one notable exception: patients with polycystic ovary syndrome.

Polycystic ovary syndrome

A diagnosis of polycystic ovary syndrome (PCOS) is made if other causes of the symptoms the patient is having are ruled out and at least two of the following three criteria are met:

1. Irregular or infrequent periods.
2. A scan showing polycystic ovaries.
3. A blood test showing high levels of 'male hormones' such as testosterone *or* just the signs of excess male hormones, like facial hair growth and acne – even if the blood test is normal.

Even in diagnosing PCOS, the blood hormone levels are not incredibly useful because in most cases they are normal.

I have actually never in my career thus far done a hormone blood test in a female acne patient and I reckon I probably never will. I have, however, diagnosed PCOS many times through clinical examination and the patient's history and have referred them to the correct specialist to confirm the diagnosis and jointly manage the patient with me to optimise their skin and health in general.

SKINTELLIGENT FACT:

Why you get spots when you get stressed

I get questions like this all the time from patients and sometimes I am lucky enough to be able to find a plausible answer. One of the underlying causes for the development of acne spots is 'sebaceous gland overactivity' – in other words, the oil glands in facial skin producing more oil than is necessary for healthy skin. The sebaceous gland function is under the influence of lots of different hormones including androgens, insulin-like growth factor and corticotropin-releasing hormone. One study showed that the increased levels of cortisol in your body as part of your stress response can increase lipid synthesis by the sebaceous glands in the skin, resulting in more oil secretion and potentially more acne.[39]

Acne in pregnancy and breastfeeding

If you get acne in pregnancy or when you are breastfeeding, it can be treated, but not as efficiently or effectively as when you aren't pregnant or breastfeeding. I think it is super important to treat acne during these times in a woman's life because it is meant to be a time of joy and happiness; and having spots can really hamper that.

The only safe options to use in pregnancy are topical benzoyl peroxide and topical azelaic acid (see pages 168 and 150). From the second trimester onwards (including after birth and while breastfeeding), for more severe acne, oral antibiotics such as erythromycin and azithromycin are safe as well. This is one time when chemical peels with glycolic or alpha-hydroxy acids may be of some help for mild acne.[40]

ATROPHIC ACNE SCARS

Atrophic acne scars are 'indented' areas of the skin where inflammation has caused damage to the collagen and elastin in the dermis. There are three types:

1. boxcar
2. ice-pick
3. rolling

Light reflects off the scars, creating shadows, and that's what makes them noticeable. Though very difficult to treat, the method with the most success is anything that physically smooths the skin surface. The gold standard is 'fractional ablative CO_2 laser resurfacing' combined with other physical treatments like subcision (using a special type of needle to break up the scar tissue directly beneath the scars, which may be pulling them down and causing the 'divot' you see in your skin), the use of high-strength peels and even punch excision (using a tiny, round-shaped apple-corer-type device) of individual scars. I counsel my patients that we are aiming for a 50 per cent improvement in skin smoothness and that repeated treatments will be needed. To improve the appearance of this type of acne scarring takes a lot of time, effort and patience.

We know that acne scars (of all types) are caused by inflammatory acne lesions that are not treated effectively or efficiently. Therefore, the best way to prevent acne scars is with effective treatment and prevention of acne.

WHEN ACNE ISN'T 'ACNE'

'Fungal' acne

A surprisingly large number of people seem to think that they have fungal acne if their acne does not respond to anti-acne cosmetic skincare products or oral antibiotics. 'Fungal' acne is actually an 'acneiform' (looks like acne, but isn't) skin rash that is caused by an overgrowth of the *Malassezia* yeast that is normally present on the skin. It is also called *Pityrosporum* folliculitis. The rash develops either due to a blockage of the hair follicle or a disturbance of the normal skin microbiome (like due to the prolonged use of antibiotics in the treatment of acne – by prolonged I mean years!). *Malassezia* lives in the sebaceous glands in the skin because it feeds off sebum.

But it doesn't look like acne vulgaris. The rash consists of very itchy, small (1–2mm) monomorphic (all the same size) follicular papules and pustules, and not just on the face: most patients also get these little bumps on the back, arms, chest and neck. And when it happens on the face, the bumps tend to occur on the chin and sides of the face, as opposed to acne vulgaris, which happens in the middle of the face.

It is more common in people with oily skin, who live in hot, humid climates, who sweat a lot, and in men. Those on immunosuppression are more at risk. Importantly, it does not improve with standard acne vulgaris treatment and that is one big clue to the diagnosis. But it is worth remembering that acne vulgaris and *Malassezia* folliculitis can coexist in anywhere from 12.2 to 27 per cent of cases.[41]

To confirm the diagnosis, you need a sample to be taken from a deep follicle; as the yeast lives on skin anyway, a skin scraping won't confirm the diagnosis.

Treatment involves taking oral antifungal tablets. Topical antifungals are not helpful because they don't penetrate deep enough into the hair follicle where the culprit yeast overgrowth lives, though they can be used alongside the tablets or even as maintenance in patients who get recurrent episodes. Itraconazole is an antifungal that may be specifically suitable for this condition and has been found to be more effective than other antifungal medicines.[42]

Exogeneous acne

In most people, acne vulgaris is a hormone-driven skin disease; it has very little, if anything, to do with what *you do* to your skin yourself. However, there is a separate category of what we call 'acneiform' eruptions (facial skin disease that looks very similar to acne but are due to external things), and it's called exogenous acne. The two most common forms of exogenous acne are acne cosmetica (acne due to the use of cosmetic products – see page 66) and acne mechanica (acne due to irritation and friction).[43] Exogenous acne generally has a very specific pattern that makes it distinct from standard acne vulgaris. With acne cosmetica, patients have comedones with few if any papules or pustules; this is extremely rare now because cosmetic manufacturers know not to include well-known comedogenic ingredients in standard formulations.[44] Acne mechanica was first described in American football players who developed acne in areas that were in contact with football helmets and shoulder pads.[45] This type of acne is characterised mainly by inflammatory papules and pustules (as opposed to predominantly non-inflammatory comedones) and is thought to be due to trauma or friction to the skin, which causes epidermal injury and results in inflammation in and around the hair follicle, leading to acne. The same type of mechanical acne can be triggered by microdermabrasion, the use of facial scrubs and the vigorous massage of a facial treatment.[46]

SKINTELLIGENT FACT:

The truth about chocolate and acne

There are two studies that have specifically looked at the effect of chocolate on acne vulgaris. The first followed a group of 25 acne-prone men over 4 weeks. Each subject consumed 25g of 99 per cent dark chocolate a day. The study found a statistically significant increase in comedones and inflammatory papules as early as two weeks into the study.[47] The second looked at the impact of both chocolate bars and jelly beans on the worsening or onset of acne.[48] They found that the chocolate bar resulted in worse acne than the jelly beans.

This looks like pretty convincing evidence that eating chocolate causes acne, right? Well, not really. The main issue with both of these studies is that chocolate is loaded with saturated fat and sugar (even the 99 per cent dark type). Another study showed that intake of full-fat dairy products was associated with moderate-to-severe acne, so the worsening of acne in the dark chocolate study is confounded by the saturated fat.[49] Sugar triggers insulin secretion and we know that both chronic and acute hyperinsulinaemia (high levels of insulin in the blood) increase levels of insulin-like growth factor 1 (IGF-1), which in turn stimulates tissue growth, including growth of the hair follicle shaft and the sebaceous gland, potentially leading to acne (and hirsutism – increased male pattern hair growth in women). We have also seen that IGF-1 stimulates skin cell (keratinocyte) proliferation in the follicle, which could also trigger acne.[50]

The story around food and acne is constantly evolving and changing. Most of the research is pointing towards insulin and insulin-like growth factor as the main culprits. Insulin in the bloodstream is increased directly because of sugar intake but also potentially via the anabolic steroids and testosterone found in industrially produced milk and dairy products. Acne is at its core a hormonally driven disease. How this works is most likely going to be a very complex pathway involving multiple inflammatory and hormone pathways, some yet to be discovered.

From a practical viewpoint, try to cut down on processed foods and carbohydrates as much as possible because, though there is no good evidence that these foods cause or worsen acne, eating a healthy diet is not harmful and could on balance potentially help. Importantly for any avid coffee drinkers, there is no clinical evidence that caffeine or coffee cause or worsen acne.

ENLARGED PORES

Facial pores are the visible openings on the skin surface of hair follicles. Each and every hair on your face has a connected oil gland, and together this structure is known as the pilosebaceous unit. We all have facial pores and they should definitely be there, but enlarged pores are a problem for many people because they are, well, large and visible.

Skin pores are classified into three types, depending on size:

1. 'Visible skin pores', which are 0.1–0.6mm wide.
2. 'Enlarged skin pores', which are 0.3–0.6mm wide.
3. 'Blackhead embedded skin pores', which are exactly as the name suggests – pores that are 'black' due to the accumulation of skin cells exposed to the air.

However, we still don't know exactly what causes pores to become visible and therefore there are no great treatments yet to make them smaller. So far, the main culprits leading to enlarged pores are thought to be the following:

1. The thicker the hair sitting in the follicle, the larger the pore.
2. The more sebum produced, the larger the pore.
3. The older you get and the more sun shines on your face, the bigger your pores become.[51]

In women during the menstrual cycle, the sebum output level is significantly higher than at other times and pore size is larger in the ovulation phase. We know that ovulation begins with a surge in luteinising hormone (LH) and follicle-stimulating hormone (FSH) levels, and progesterone levels also start to increase. Note that normal levels of oestrogen have very little, if any, effect on regulating oil glands. Most enlarged pores are on the nose and the cheek in the middle of your face. This is also where the most oil is produced on the face.

And, of course, ageing and sun exposure cause changes in elasticity in the skin, leading to loss of some of the structural support that the dermis provides for the hair follicle, which may lead to sagging and enlargement of the hair follicle opening. In short, there is decreased elasticity supporting the structure of your pores as you age![52]

There are tons of products on the market that claim to reduce pore size (like clay masks, pore strips, scrubs, primers . . .), but, unfortunately, they don't really work (as you may have discovered yourself) and there are no evidence-based studies to support their use. As I often say, 'pores don't have doors – you can't open and close them'.

So, what can you do that might actually help?

If you are looking to reduce the size of your pores, top of the list of possibilities sits oral isotretinoin (see page 179), as it is the most effective medicine to drastically reduce oil production. Other oral treatments include anti-androgens like spironolactone and the combined oral contraceptive pill (see page 175). Studies indicate that these types of treatments can reduce oil secretion by anywhere from 12.5 to 65 per cent.[53] Injecting botulinum toxin (such as Botox) into the dermis has also been reported to improve pore size (see page 234).[54] These are all treatments usually prescribed by a dermatologist.

In terms of improving skin elasticity, aside from the use of topical tretinoin, there are a huge variety of treatments and devices that claim they can improve skin elasticity. In my clinical practice, the gold-standard laser for improving skin texture and possibly reducing pore size is the CO_2 fractional ablative laser, which also has the strongest evidence base for safety and efficacy.

SEBACEOUS FILAMENTS ON THE NOSE

If you have ever examined the skin on your nose with a magnifying mirror, you have probably noticed little black dots, perhaps with small hairs poking out of them. If you have pinched the skin, you may have even been able to squeeze out the little black dot, only to realise that it leaves behind a tiny opening in your skin (which is a hair follicle opening), and that the little black dot is not actually a dot but rather a white-yellow worm-like structure. Patients often think these are blackheads, which they are not: blackheads are plugs at the top of a pore (a hair follicle opening on the skin). A blackhead prevents oil from escaping through the pore and it is dark because the keratin that makes it up has been oxidised through exposure to air. What is actually on your nose is a sebaceous filament – a thin, hair-like structure that lines the inside of the pore and actually helps sebum travel to the skin's surface. It isn't a plug at all.

Sebaceous filaments are most commonly found in the parts of the face that have the most oil production – so the area of the central face often referred to as the T zone (the nose, between the eyebrows, the forehead and the chin). People with oily skin tend to have more prominent sebaceous filaments. The stuff you can squeeze out is a mixture of bacteria, sebum and fragments of corneocytes. Once you have squeezed out the content of the follicle it will refill within 30 days. It is important to remember that these sebaceous filaments are actually a normal part of your skin's structure and have a purpose to being there.[55]

So what can you do about them? Not very much, unfortunately – no skincare product can get rid of sebaceous filaments and repeatedly squeezing them out can sometimes damage the skin. The only thing that may help over time is reducing the oiliness of your skin, with some of the methods mentioned above, such as oral isotretinoin.[56]

13

Rosacea

Though often misdiagnosed, rosacea has a classical appearance that is 'once seen, never forgotten'. It tends to affect both women and men, usually from their early thirties, about 5.5 per cent of the adult population and it is found predominantly in fair-skinned people, though this may be partially due to the difficulty in detecting facial redness in darker skin types.[1] There are some key signs to look out for:

- papules and pustules
- visible blood vessels
- persistent facial redness
- flushing and blushing
- thickened facial skin (mainly of the nose, but this type of change happens after many years of having rosacea)
- eye problems

The spots are usually small red bumps ('papules'), some filled with pus ('pustules' or 'papulopustules'). These spots are mainly found in the central part of the face – the nose, cheeks, chin, forehead and between the eyebrows (the glabella). The areas immediately around the eyes and mouth are not involved (which is one distinct difference with acne vulgaris). Another key distinguishing feature between acne vulgaris and rosacea is that in rosacea there are no comedones. Aside from the flushing and blushing, which can feel hot, most people don't experience a change of sensation in their skin from rosacea, though women more commonly complain of a burning sensation. The distribution of the spots tends to be symmetrical on the face, but it can be more severe on one side or even completely unilateral (one-sided).

The word rosacea comes from the Latin adjective meaning 'like roses'. The word 'acne' shouldn't really be attached to rosacea, since acne is a totally different thing, so for the sake of correctness and clarity, I refer to it simply as 'rosacea'.[2]

WHAT CAUSES ROSACEA?

There is no perfect explanation for why some people have this problem. The current favoured theory is that it is due to stress on the endoplasmic reticulum (ER), which is a transportation system inside each and every one of our cells, and it becomes dysregulated in patients with rosacea, causing a cascade of chemical and molecular changes in the skin, resulting in the signs and symptoms of rosacea that you see. Prevention of rosacea is aimed, therefore, at avoiding triggers of ER stress, and symptom therapy aims to reduce the cascade of events that ER stress sets off.

When the skin of people with rosacea is biopsied and examined under a microscope, there are some common features: sun damage is always seen, but the inflammation seen is not limited to the hair follicle unit, like it is in acne vulgaris. Rosacea is thought of as a vascular disease, meaning it has to do with an abnormality of the blood vessels in the skin. Under the microscope, the blood vessels and lymph vessels in the dermis are dilated (enlarged) with white blood cells present, indicating inflammation. The more advanced the disease, the more enlarged the vessels become. There are usually more white blood cells in the hair follicles when papules and pustules are seen on the skin.

The redness of the facial skin is generally not associated with an increase in the temperature of the skin – so the redness isn't due to increased blood flow, but rather 'pooling' of the blood in the dilated blood vessels. Flushing is a visible consequence of the temporary filling of the dilated blood vessels and the redness is due to permanent vasodilatation (enlargement or opening of blood vessels) in the dermis and below.[3] In rosacea patients, the papillary (upper) dermis is found to have many irregularly dilated capillary vessels and disorganisation of dermal connective tissue (like collagen and elastin), which does not provide the structural support that the small blood vessels that feed the skin (known as microvasculature) need. This can all be attributed to sun damage over time.

Rosacea usually starts with intermittent flushing, which gradually over time develops into persistent redness of the skin. This points to a problem with regulation of the blood vessels in the skin. Most studies also show that there is reduced water content in the stratum corneum and increased transepidermal water loss (TEWL – see page 15) in the facial skin of rosacea patients.[4] Interestingly, patients with rosacea do not produce more surface oil than non-rosacea patients, even though rosacea predominantly affects the oil-rich middle part of the face. However, there appears to be a change in the composition of the skin surface oil in patients with rosacea, which seems to be one of the underlying reasons for the disturbed stratum corneum. There is definitely a sebaceous gland dysfunction in rosacea patients that partially explains why it occurs in the first place, but also why low-dose oral isotretinoin is so effective at treating it (by reducing oil secretion) – see page 179.[5]

One common finding in people with rosacea is the presence of *Demodex folliculorum* mites. Though I appreciate this sounds terrible, these little guys are present on everyone's skin and usually do no harm. In fact, they can only survive on human skin! It is important to remember that *Demodex* mites are not the cause of rosacea, but rather a consequence of it because the other skin changes that occur make the skin of rosacea patients a great home for the mites.

Rosacea patients tend to flush and blush easily, which gets

worse with sun exposure, heat (like hot weather), a sudden change in ambient temperature, drinking hot drinks and experiencing emotional stress. It is a misconception that it is the caffeine content of beverages that cause people to flush; the specific stimulus is actually heat and caffeine itself (in trials, up to 200mg per drink) caused no flushing at all if the drink was cold.[6] The association of smoking and alcohol as well as spicy food is observed inconsistently. But one thing is for certain: patients with rosacea do flush more often and more deeply than a non-rosacea population.

Flushing and blushing in and of itself is not diagnostic of rosacea. Facial flushing is quite common in the world; children flush, as do women going through the menopause. Indeed, having a red or ruddy complexion with dilated capillaries (telangiectasia) is also not diagnostic of rosacea.

SKINTELLIGENT FACT:

Screen dermatitis

Since the late 1970s, facial skin symptoms related to chronic exposure to 'visual display units' (screens) have been mainly reported in Scandinavia. These patients were described as having rosacea-like facial skin changes, such as redness, bumps and pustules, along with symptoms of pain, itching and a heat sensation similar to sunburn. But is there a relationship between screens and a facial skin rash resembling rosacea?

Studies have found that the most common skin disease presenting in people who continuously use computer screens (like video gamers) is indeed rosacea.[7] 'Screen dermatitis' is a recognised skin disease that is believed to be due to non-irritating factors specifically found in patients with hyper-reactive ('sensitive') skin and psychosocial stress. But it has never been shown that anything coming from the screens – like electric or magnetic fields – is capable of causing these types of skin changes.

Yes, it is confusing! If you have rosacea, it's probably not your screen that is to blame, but rather the stress induced by having to use it all the time!

There are no tests to diagnosis rosacea and, recently, the diagnostic criteria for it have changed. It was previously classified by four subtypes (type 1 being 'erythematelangiectatic', type 2 being 'pustular', and so on), but this has now been changed to a 'phenotype' approach, which is based on clinical examination and the patient's history. This is great because it allows for more focused treatment.[8] The diagnosis is made with the presence of either changes to the skin of the nose (thickening of the skin due to fibrosis or enlargement of the sebaceous glands, giving the nose a bulbous appearance) or persistent, ongoing background facial redness in the middle of the face, which can get redder or more intense from time to time when the patient is exposed to various triggers.

If neither of those two features is present, the diagnosis can be made if you have any *two* of the following major features:

- flushing that is fairly regular and associated with sensations of warmth, heat, burning or pain
- the presence of little red bumps (pustules and papules)
- the presence of visible dilated capillaries or thread veins (telangiectasia), not only around the nostrils but also on the cheeks, forehead and chin[9]

Burning, stinging or dry skin that feels rough, tight, scaly or itchy is not diagnostic of rosacea.

SKINTELLIGENT TIP:

You can use topical tretinoin for anti-ageing if you have rosacea

Many patients fear using topical tretinoin if they have rosacea because they know or have heard that tretinoin can make skin red, inflamed, itchy or peel at the beginning of treatment. And many rosacea patients have very reactive skin to different products and know to avoid certain things. Clinical trial data does support the beneficial use of topical tretinoin in those with rosacea, though.[10] I generally don't use tretinoin to treat active rosacea, but once it is under control, I will start it if my patient is keen on the anti-ageing benefits. I will always start with the lowest possible strength (usually 0.01 per cent), using it alternate nights only, and we build it up slowly. Some rosacea patients (myself included) experience irritation and increased redness if used daily; if this is you, don't worry, you can still get the benefits of tretinoin even at a low strength and used only a few times a week. Just be consistent.

TREATMENTS FOR PAPULES AND PUSTULES

There are three topical treatments approved for the treatment of the papules and pustules of rosacea: metronidazole was the first one (0.75 per cent or 1 per cent) and is still considered the cornerstone of topical treatment. It is applied once or twice daily and works as an anti-inflammatory agent. It is generally very well-tolerated by patients and causes no irritation. Azelaic acid (15 or 20 per cent) is also an anti-inflammatory agent for rosacea (see page 150), also applied twice daily. It can cause skin irritation with redness and burning in the first two weeks of treatment. The most recently approved treatment is Ivermectin (1 per cent) cream, which is both an anti-inflammatory and an anti-parasite drug that kills the *Demodex* mite in the skin. It is applied once daily at night. It can also cause skin irritation with burning, itching and dry skin, and can worsen redness considerably.[11]

Combining topical treatments with anti-inflammatory tetracycline antibiotics (like doxycycline) is standard first-line treatment for most rosacea patients. If that combination is not effective after 3–6 months, low-dose oral isotretinoin is a very successful treatment. Low-dose means anywhere from 5 to 20mg a day and is considered slightly more effective than doxycycline. Of course, all the same guidelines apply in the use of isotretinoin in women of childbearing age due to its ability to cause birth defects (see page 183).[12] In my clinical experience, not only is low-dose isotretinoin the most effective treatment for the papules and pustules of rosacea, it can also improve generalised redness.

TREATMENTS FOR FLUSHING AND GENERALISED REDNESS

The flushing and redness of rosacea are probably the most challenging to treat. The first step is to do your best to avoid your triggers – sun exposure being the most important one. People with rosacea have 'hyper-reactive' skin – which is partially due to a damaged skin barrier allowing penetration of irritants, but also already inflamed skin is more prone to developing reactions to irritants. One study showed that rosacea patients are more likely to react to allergens in cosmetic skincare products than the general population.[13] So, one great way to reduce redness and flushing is to scale back on skincare products and use only the most basic, simple cleanser and moisturiser that you like and can afford (good old Vaseline fits the bill again here!).

In 2013, the FDA approved topical brimonidine (0.33 per cent) gel as a once-daily treatment for facial redness (it is also licensed for this in the UK). Brimonidine tartrate is a 'vasoconstrictor', meaning it closes the vessels in the dermis and therefore takes away the redness. It works within 20 minutes of application and usually lasts for up to 12 hours. About 20 per cent of patients who use it experience 'rebound' redness after it wears off or with long-term use. Another FDA-approved cream (not currently available in the UK) that does a similar thing is oxymetazoline (1 per cent). It is supposed to cause less of a redness rebound than brimonidine, but it has not been studied long-term yet or directly compared to brimonidine in a clinical trial. In my clinical experience, patients find these types of creams useful if they need to control their redness for a special event, but most do not use them daily. They also don't help control flushing or any of the other signs or symptoms of rosacea.[14]

Yet another option for background redness is laser treatment, which is discussed in detail on page 212.

Neurotoxin

It is hypothesised that some of the problems of rosacea are due to a 'neuron-mediated' vascular dysfunction, which means that nerves in the skin affect how much blood flows into it by acting directly on blood vessels. Neurotoxin (such as Botox) works by blocking the release of acetylcholine (ACH), which is one of the neurotransmitters that signals changes in blood vessel diameter (for more on this, see page 234). Based on this, the use of neurotoxin is a suggested approach for the management of the flushing and persistent redness of rosacea. Instead of injecting into the muscle, which would be the technique for treating wrinkles, for redness the neurotoxin is injected into the dermis (intradermally) and in very small quantities, to minimise the risk of it affecting the underlying muscles. The claimed effects of these 'micro' injections into, for example, the cheek area, include a reduction in oil production, decreased papules and pustules, reduced flushing in the treated area and an overall reduction in facial redness. (Neurotoxin potentially also blocks the activity of ACH on sebocytes – the cells of the oil glands.)[15]

Two randomised controlled trials of the use of neurotoxin in the treatment of the redness of rosacea found conflicting results (in one study it worked well, in the other it didn't), but both had a small number of subjects, which makes it hard to draw any meaningful conclusions.[16]

One study recently combined treatment with a pulsed dye laser and intradermal neurotoxin injection in 20 rosacea patients with redness and flushing – the first study of its kind. Researchers found that there was a high level of patient satisfaction with this combination and also an improvement in the objective measurement of redness, with few side effects.[17] Another study combined the use of neurotoxin with another ablative laser. The study only included 16 patients with a short 6-month follow-up period only, but outcomes were good.[18]

The bottom line: The verdict is still out on whether neurotoxin can be safe and effective for the treatment of facial redness and flushing, though in a recent systematic review, all patients saw an improvement in the signs and symptoms of rosacea with minimal short-term side effects.[19]

Carvedilol

Another option for facial flushing and redness is the use of carvedilol, a beta-blocker, which is a class of drug normally used to lower blood pressure. It is also often used to treat symptoms of anxiety. Carvedilol has been trialled at a very low dose in patients with normal blood pressure to reduce flushing and redness. It is thought to work by causing constriction or narrowing of some of the blood vessels in the skin. The dose ranges from 6.25 to 12.5mg twice daily (for comparison, when carvedilol is used to treat high blood pressure it is 50mg twice daily) and has been found to be effective.[20] I have used this in patients, and it has worked very well.

FACIAL TELANGIECTASIA

There are two interconnecting 'highways' of blood vessels in the skin. One runs through the middle of the dermis, at the junction of the papillary (upper) and reticular (lower) dermis. The other one is deeper down, at the junction between the dermis and the fat tissue beneath and has larger blood vessels in it. The lymphatic vessels and the nerves run alongside both sets of blood vessels.[21]

Telangiectasia are the fine thread veins that are commonly seen on the noses and cheeks of fair-skinned people. You may refer to them as 'broken capillaries', but this is a misnomer because they are, in fact, widened or 'dilated' capillaries and not broken at all. The blood vessels in the skin live in the dermis and telangiectasia are the manifestation of massive dilation of the most superficial capillaries in the papillary (upper) dermis. They occur as we age as a result of weakening of the wall of the blood vessel, due to changes in the supportive connective tissue surrounding the vessel, secondary to chronic sun exposure.

You are most likely to develop telangiectasia if you have fair skin and you smoke. Getting older is also a major cause. Females tend to have them more often than males, and if you sunburn easily, you will probably have more as well. Smoking is by far the biggest risk factor, and this is not hugely surprising considering that smoking is one of the most important lifestyle factors causing premature skin ageing. Smoking, of course, causes DNA damage, but also damages the elastin in the dermis (as it does in the lungs), which harms the supportive structures around the capillaries and therefore allows them to dilate more than they should.[22] Physical trauma or damage to the skin can also lead to telangiectasia, especially along stitch lines from facial surgery.

Treatment options

Though telangiectasia are considered a normal part of skin ageing, many people (including myself!) don't like them and want to get rid of them. And this is where the challenge starts.

Unfortunately, there is no skin cream that will fix facial telangiectasia. However, both laser/light devices and hand cautery can be used to attempt to get rid of them.

The main problem with the treatment of telangiectasia is that treatments need to be repeated, anywhere from six to ten or more individual treatments spaced about four weeks apart – and probably maintenance treatments will be required periodically forever. How often will depend on each individual patient's response to treatment, how severe their condition is and ongoing exposure to UV light (which is inevitable for most people, no matter how hard you try to avoid it!). I have found that a combination of laser or light treatment with hand cautery gives the best outcome, but treatments need to be continued. All treatments can be irritating to skin, especially that of patients with rosacea, so making sure your active rosacea is under control is important before undertaking any of these treatments. Also, it's worth bearing in mind that all of them have some level of recovery time after the treatment itself; anything that destroys a vessel will almost certainly leave behind some bruising (known as purpura), which usually takes up to 14 days to completely resolve.

Lasers

The lasers used to get rid of telangiectasia include the following:

- KTP (532nm)
- pulse dye (595nm)
- Alexandrite (755nm)
- diode (810nm)
- Nd:YAG (1064nm)

Though they each represent a different wavelength of light, they work by the light being attracted to the haemoglobin in the blood vessel and damaging the vessel wall, therefore causing destruction of the vessel. Intense Pulsed Light (IPL) works in a similar way, but is not a laser in that it is a spectrum of wavelengths rather than just one.

Lasers in the 500–600nm wavelength are favoured for telangiectasia because they are highly absorbed by haemoglobin (blood) and not so well by anything else, like pigment in the skin (melanin). However, they can still cause pigmentation problems in darker-skinned people. The infrared range of lasers (800–1100nm) can also work for haemoglobin and are less absorbed by melanin, making them safer for darker skinned people. Longer wavelength lasers penetrate deeper into the skin, with the Nd:YAG laser being the deepest penetrating laser in human tissue. Generally, most practitioners will use a KTP or pulse dye laser for finer vessels, and for anything larger than 1mm in diameter, the Nd:YAG is more suitable.[23] There is still no agreement on which laser is best and, in my experience, the best laser for you is probably the one your doctor knows and understands best and has had the most experience with.

Hand cautery

Hand cautery, also known as electrosurgery, is a procedure in which a small needle is applied on the skin along the length of the telangiectasia or at the root of the vessel, and then an electric current is used to 'seal' the vessel. Because it is a monopolar current, people with pacemakers or implantable cardio-defibrillators cannot have this treatment. I have only ever come across one published study of this technique (though it is quite extensively used in clinical practice). In the study, 88 per cent of 25 patients had complete resolution of their facial telangiectasia with hand cautery, with 20 per cent only requiring one treatment.[24] The treatment was performed mainly around the nose, but also on the chin and the cheek. The lesions around the nose were the most responsive. Indeed, in my own clinical practice, I have found that the juicier vessels on the nose, around the nostrils, respond best to treatment and the finer ones on the cheek and chin often only partially improve or do not respond.

14

Dermatitis

D ermatitis is a general term that refers to anything that causes skin irritation in the form of itchy, red, flaky skin. There are many things that can cause dermatitis and in this chapter I am going to cover the most common forms that affect the face that I see in my clinic every day.

PERIORAL DERMATITIS

One of the most common skin problems I see in my female patients is perioral dermatitis. Indeed, 90 per cent of those affected are females between the ages of 20 and 45.[1] It has quite a striking appearance: the patients develop small red bumps (papules) and tiny pus-filled spots (micropustules) in a distinct pattern affecting the area around the nostril, nasolabial fold (the line between your cheek and your upper lip) and along the chin. The lip border is never affected. It can also affect the skin around the eyes, but not the eyelash line itself. The little bumps are monomorphic (all the same size), there are no comedones (to distinguish it from acne vulgaris) and the background skin on which the bumps sit is red. The rash can be a little itchy or flaky at times.[2]

Typically, the patient has been given or used a topical steroid to treat the rash; this is the incorrect treatment as it will clear the rash for a day or two, but when the steroid is stopped it will come back again immediately. This gets the patient into a bad cycle where they then use the steroid again to clear it, but immediately upon stopping it comes back, often worse than it was and then the patient feels compelled to use the steroid again, continuing the cycle.

We don't really know what the true underlying cause of perioral dermatitis is, but it is associated with the use of topical steroids on the face, as well as nasal or inhaled steroids, fluorinated toothpaste, dental fillings and even chewing gum! Sun exposure can also bring it on, as can lipstick and emotional stress. In my patients I find that the most common cause is the overuse of irritating cosmetic products or using too many products at once (like multiple skincare products being layered and then make-up like foundation and powder added on top).

But rest assured, perioral dermatitis can be simply and effectively treated. The first thing to do is stop or avoid all potential triggers – and that includes all cosmetic skincare products. I often get my patients to literally stop everything, including any topical steroid creams and wearing make-up, if possible, just during the first week or two of treatment while the rash clears up. I advise cleansing the skin with water only and using only Vaseline on the rest of the face (no surprise there!).

My first-line treatment is a combination of oral antibiotics (usually lymecycline or erythromycin) as well as either topical tacrolimus, pimecrolimus or metronidazole gel. Most patients improve rapidly with these simple steps and the perioral dermatitis generally doesn't come back!

SEBORRHEIC DERMATITIS

Seborrheic dermatitis affects skin in oil-rich areas of the face and body (the scalp, around the nose and eyebrows, the chest) and makes the areas red and scaly. The scale is generally yellow and greasy. It is considered the same condition as cradle cap that happens in infants (though cradle cap is managed differently!). Seborrheic dermatitis is more common in men than in women, affects 1–3 per cent of adults and is more common in people over the age of 50.[3] It is often associated with an itchy scalp and dandruff.

This condition was first connected with *Malassezia* yeast in 1874 by Louis-Charles Malassez (hence the name) – he suggested that the rash is an exaggerated inflammatory response to the presence of the yeast on the skin. *Malassezia* is a normal part of the skin flora, and it feeds off sebum on the skin (see page 195). There is a link as the rash occurs in the oil-rich areas of the skin and it often improves with anti-yeast agents (for example, the use of ketoconazole shampoo to treat dandruff), but how exactly this yeast stimulates or induces the red, scaly rash of seborrheic dermatitis is not known.

Other recent suggestions have been that seborrheic dermatitis is a form of psoriasis that occurs on the face. Psoriasis is a condition in which well-defined, red plaques covered in thick, silvery scale appear on the body, especially the knees and elbows. It is called a 'hyperproliferative' disease because in psoriasis the stratum corneum 'builds up' more quickly than it sheds, resulting in the thickened plaques of skin (see page 22).[4]

My preferred way to treat seborrheic dermatitis on the face is with topical tacrolimus or pimecrolimus, which are non-steroid prescription anti-inflammatory creams. For scalp involvement, the best treatment I have found is a compounded shampoo containing ketoconazole, salicylic acid and a mild steroid. I also often use a moderate steroid combined with salicylic or glycolic acid as a scalp application to clear the scale and reduce the itching and inflammation. After initial daily or twice-daily use of treatment, most patients find their condition completely resolves. Maintenance of clearance usually involves using the treatments once or twice a week only.

FACIAL ECZEMA

'Eczema' is a general term referring to skin that is itchy, red, dry and cracked. It comes from the Greek for 'to boil over'. Dermatitis is a synonym for eczema and is also a general term meaning 'inflammation of the skin'. Eczematous dermatitis is one of the most common problems we see in dermatology. Some people also refer to it as 'atopic dermatitis' (atopy is a word used to describe a person's general tendency to develop allergies to things, like in asthma or hay fever).

Many people have dry skin on their face at some point from one thing or another, but eczema or dermatitis is different because of the severity of the dryness and its associated symptoms. On the face, it generally affects the eyelid skin and the skin around the mouth, though it can affect the entire face.

With isolated facial or eyelid eczema, the most important thing to rule out is whether it is an allergic contact dermatitis. This is eczema on the face due to an allergy (a sensitivity) to something that has been or is being applied to the skin or coming into contact with the skin. The most common contact allergy in general (but not specifically for the face) is due to nickel; if you have ever had itchy red skin around your earlobes or neck after wearing certain pieces of jewellery you probably have a nickel allergy. 'Fake' jewellery (not pure gold or silver, for example) often has nickel added to it. If you come into contact with the nickel-containing jewellery and it stays in contact with your skin for a few hours, you will develop eczema in that area.

Whenever I have a patient with a contact dermatitis due to a skincare product, the thing they most often say is that the dermatitis suddenly appeared, and they had not changed anything in their skincare routine or the products they use. It is possible to develop a contact allergy to the same product after using it for many years; you can develop a sensitivity to an allergen you were not previously allergic to and often the formulation of your favourite products can be changed without you realising it (Big Skincare is at it again!).

It is extremely common to have an allergic contact dermatitis to cosmetics and skincare. The eyelids are frequently involved with common sources of allergen including shampoos, conditioners, facial cleansers, make-up removers, mascara, nail polish, acrylic nails, make-up sponges, eyelash curlers and allergens transferred from hands.[5] When it comes to eyelid dermatitis, the most common cause of it is seborrheic dermatitis (in one study, 46.3 per cent had seborrheic dermatitis and 35.2 per cent had contact dermatitis).[6] However, when other parts of the face were affected aside from just the eyelids, allergic contact dermatitis was the most frequent cause. It is important to note that contact dermatitis of the eyelids and the area around the eye is primarily caused by cosmetics applied to the hair, face or fingernails rather than the eyelid itself. Remember that the eyelid skin is occluded while the eye is open – meaning chemicals are 'trapped' in that area – and the thin stratum corneum and epidermis of the eyelid mean it is more susceptible to irritation. The reason why shampoo and facial cleansers can cause eyelid dermatitis is because when you wash your hair or your face, the products often 'gather' in your eyelid creases and many people don't rinse them away properly. This allows the product to have prolonged contact with the eyelid skin, causing a reaction to occur. The sides of the face or neck can also develop dermatitis this way, in a 'rinse-off' pattern.[7]

If a patient presents with isolated facial eczema, the first thing I do is take a thorough history and examine the face (and the body – including the hands!) carefully and try to work out what type of product could be driving the problem. If I suspect a contact allergy, patch testing is the only way to be certain what chemical is the problem. This involves putting small discs ('patches') of specific known allergens on a patient's back for up to 72 hours and seeing if eczema develops where the patches are placed. If it does, then that usually indicates that specific chemical is the culprit.[8]

Once the culprit is known, then avoidance of that chemical is the key to clearing up the eczema. My preferred treatment for facial eczema is non-steroid anti-inflammatory topical treatments like tacrolimus or pimecrolimus.

Irritant dermatitis can also occur on the face, and it is something I see very often in my clinical practice, especially in young women who like to use lots of skincare and make-up products. This is not a true allergy, but rather a hypersensitivity to products in general. In patients who experience this, they find all cosmetics or products applied to the face produce itching, burning or stinging. Why this develops is not completely understood, but the way to correct it is by total avoidance of all facial cosmetics for a prolonged period of time (like six months to a year). This includes not allowing shampoo and conditioner to touch the face, as well as avoidance of all moisturisers, surfactants and colour cosmetics. I usually only allow my patients with this problem to use water to cleanse and very bland emollients (Vaseline again!) and sometimes powder foundations, but that's it.

15

Melasma and Facial Hyperpigmentation

Melasma is not a 'cosmetic' problem – it's an actual skin disease: I define a skin disease as anything that represents an abnormality of the skin, when it doesn't look the way it should. Melasma is too much pigment in the skin and we still don't really know the exact cause, though fluctuating levels of female hormones are theorised as being the culprit – for example, during pregnancy, by taking the combined contraceptive pill or during perimenopause or menopause.

Unfortunately, Big Skincare is trying to make you believe that melasma can be treated with a set of over-the-counter cleansers, serums and moisturisers you can purchase at your local beauty counter or 'medispa'. And that is categorically and absolutely a lie. **No over-the-counter cosmetic product or series of products will treat your melasma.** It is a skin disease and needs a medical treatment. Melasma is one of those skin conditions that you should see a consultant or board-certified dermatologist about. Do not DIY this with the help of the 'friendly' ladies at the beauty counter or a beautician. You will waste tons of money and not get anywhere.

And please don't ask, 'What about kojic acid? Glycolic acid? Arbutin? Vitamin C? Niacinamide? I was told those work really well for pigmentation.' They don't – it's all a lie to sell you products.

TREATMENTS THAT WORK FOR MELASMA

First, I get my patients with melasma to stop using all cosmetic skincare except the absolute basics. Then I start them on a compounded prescription product of tretinoin, hydroquinone and usually a teeny bit of hydrocortisone (a mild steroid cream), and give them extremely specific instructions on how to use the product. The tretinoin helps to prevent the hydroquinone from oxidising and temporarily thins the stratum corneum to allow for the hydroquinone to better penetrate the skin, and the hydrocortisone helps reduce the irritation that may be caused by both the tretinoin and the hydroquinone.

I know that many people have concerns about using hydroquinone, but when used appropriately under medical supervision it is safe and effective.[1] I usually start patients on 0.025 per cent tretinoin combined with hydroquinone 4–10 per cent and hydrocortisone 0.5 per cent (though the exact strengths depend on the patient). This is the night-time treatment. For severe melasma or pigmentation, I often add in a morning hydroquinone cream as well.

The aim of treatment is to get the melasma to clear as quickly as possible. Once adequate clearance is reached, I start to reduce the hydroquinone concentration in the cream and increase the tretinoin, as tolerated.

Often, I add in oral tranexamic acid (TXA) if there is no reason why the patient cannot take it, like a history of blood clots. TXA is a medicine that is used to control bleeding by helping your blood clot; in the UK you can buy it from any pharmacy if you suffer from heavy periods. Since 1979, it has been used to treat melasma. See page 227 for more detailed information about TXA.

I also counsel my patients about strict sun-avoidance tactics. And then we wait. There is no overnight magic; no five-step skincare regime costing hundreds of pounds or series of laser treatments. Correct diagnosis, an evidence-based management plan, consistency and patience – that's the magic melasma treatment combo.

THE MOST COMMON QUESTIONS I GET ASKED ABOUT MELASMA TREATMENT

Can triple combination cream cause telangiectasia?

This is something I see occasionally with my melasma patients; they use the treatment, their melasma improves and they notice that they have telangiectasia (fine thread veins) on their cheeks or nose or the area that previously had melasma patches. Patients often come back to me saying that they think the tretinoin caused the dilated capillaries to appear.

Chronic sun exposure, genetics and intrinsic ageing cause the dilated capillaries that we call telangiectasia to appear, and they are much more common in people with lighter skin colour (see page 210). Tretinoin does not cause them or make them worse if they are already present. One study showed via immunohistology that there was an increase in blood vessels, allowing for more blood to flow to the dermis (increased vascularity) after 48 weeks of treatment with tretinoin 0.05 and 0.025 per cent.[2] Increased vascularity in the dermis may be an important aspect of tretinoin treatment of intrinsic and photoageing of the skin because the positive anti-ageing changes require increased blood flow, but they do not cause telangiectasia to appear on the skin.

There might be a subtype of melasma, however, called 'telangiectatic' melasma. This was first described in the medical literature in 2010, with a report of four unique patients where melasma appeared in conjunction with underlying telangiectasia.[3] Prior to that, it was believed that melasma was associated with telangiectasia for various reasons – like pregnancy, the use of topical steroids, sun damage or underlying rosacea coexisting with melasma. In the report, the four patients described had none of these related problems. They were treated with standard triple combination therapy for 12 weeks successfully, uncovering the underlying telangiectasia. Usually, the telangiectasia can be seen with a dermatoscope through the melasma patches on the face. I now specifically examine for the presence of telangiectasia prior to starting patients on treatment so they are aware of what to expect to see when their pigmentation clears.

Is it safe to have steroids in the treatment for melasma?

Triple combination cream containing hydroquinone, tretinoin and a mild topical steroid is the gold-standard treatment for melasma and facial hyperpigmentation. The low-potency steroid helps enhance the depigmenting activity of hydroquinone because topical steroids are known to also have a mild skin-lightening effect on their own. The tretinoin causes the pigment granules in the keratinocytes (skin cells) to disperse and speeds up how quickly cells of the epidermis renew so the pigment can be lost more rapidly.[4] The steroid works to balance the initial thinning effect of tretinoin on the stratum corneum, while the tretinoin overrides the potential thinning effects of the steroid while not having any impact on its ability to reduce its anti-inflammatory effect.

Despite this combination being an FDA- and MHRA-approved treatment for melasma, patients are often still concerned about long-term use of even weak or low-potency topical steroids, but research has found no evidence of thinning (atrophy) of the epidermis or dermis at any point, though there was a marked reduction in epidermal melanin in keeping with a clinical improvement in melasma.[5]

The bottom line: It is safe to have a low-potency steroid in triple combination cream for the treatment of melasma.

Is 'dermal' melasma a real thing?

The majority of my melasma patients have seen countless other healthcare professionals for treatment before coming to me. One thing I hear very often is that their previous treatments failed because they have 'dermal' melasma – at least that is what they have been told as the reason why the treatment did not work. This is odd to me because there is no such thing as 'dermal' melasma – this is an archaic term that has been shown to be incorrect.[6]

One study looked at melasma facial skin compared to normal skin under a microscope.[7] The findings are super interesting:

- Both areas of skin showed evidence of chronic sun damage.
- Melasma skin had more melanin (pigment) in the entire epidermis than the non-melasma skin, in which the pigment was mainly only in the bottom of the epidermis where it normally should be.
- Melasma skin has more melanocytes and melanin in the epidermis (see page 23) than non-melasma skin.
- There was no significant difference in the quantity of melanophages in the dermis of melasma versus non-melasma skin, indicating that there is no 'true' dermal melasma type. (Melanophages are white blood cells that remove melanin from the skin – they are normally found in the dermis where they 'eat up' melanin that gets into the dermis because generally it is not supposed to be there!)

Melasma is epidermal hyperpigmentation. The melanocytes in the epidermis of people with melasma seem to make a lot more melanin in the patches of melasma and this happens by the action of the enzyme tyrosinase converting tyrosine into melanin. 'Deactivating' this enzyme is the key to clearing melasma and that is what hydroquinone does (see page 133).

Should you have a peel to treat your melasma?

If you have melasma, you have probably searched online to find some treatment ideas. One of the most well-marketed treatments for pigmentation is an in-office peel that goes by a variety of brand names and costs from £600 per treatment. The peel is a mix of cosmetic 'anti-pigment' ingredients like kojic acid, phytic acid, ascorbic acid, arbutin, mandelic acid and glycolic acid. The marketing will tell you that it should reduce pigmentation by 95 per cent after 30 days. But does it work? Does it last? And is it worth the money (and the recovery time)?

After reviewing several melasma treatments, I found very little high-quality evidence to support the use of chemical peels in the treatment of melasma.[8] In my 'treatment ladder', I list it as third-line and only in combination with first-line treatments.

Chemical peels are not anywhere near as effective as the marketing material may have you believe and, if some improvement is seen, it is short-lived. Unless you are going to commit to doing one of these peels every 1–2 months, possibly forever, they are not a realistic or (for most) financially feasible way of clearing melasma in the long term. The same applies to the use of lasers for melasma (even the Pico laser!).

Don't believe the marketing and please don't get tricked into parting with possibly thousands of pounds of cash for one of these peels.

SKINTELLIGENT TIP:

Heat* does not make melasma worse

(*hot showers, saunas, intense exercise, cooking over a hot stove, etc.)
I still can't figure out where this concept has come from - that exposing one's face to a heat source can

somehow worsen melasma. It's not something I have ever come across clinically during my career to date and it is not mentioned as a trigger anywhere in the scientific literature. But it is something that patients ask me about all the time.

Several papers list the trigger factors for melasma as the following:[9]

- chronic sun (UV) exposure
- genetics
- female sex hormones
- inflammatory processes in the skin (like acne or eczema)

None of them mention heat as a trigger.

The bottom line: If you have melasma, you can take a hot shower, hang out in a sauna, sweat through an intense work-out and even cook over a hot stove, without the fear of making your melasma worse.

How do tranexamic acid (TXA) tablets work to treat melasma?

If you have ever suffered from heavy periods, you may have taken TXA to lighten them because it works to stop the breakdown of a protein called fibrin, and fibrin is one of the main components of a blood clot. Hence, TXA reduces blood flow.

It was first used in the treatment of melasma in 1979.[10] Below is a step-by-step explanation of how we think TXA works to lighten melasma:[11]

1. Plasmin found in keratinocytes induces the production of both arachidonic acid and alpha-melanocyte-stimulating hormone.
2. Arachidonic acid and alpha-melanocyte-stimulating hormone stimulate the production of melanin (skin pigment) by melanocytes, which can lead to melasma.
3. Plasminogen activator is required to make plasmin do what it does in the keratinocytes.
4. Plasminogen activator has lysine-binding sites on it – these sites need to be stimulated to activate the activator to then go on to get plasmin to do its thing.
5. TXA is a synthetic derivative of the amino acid lysine – it looks like lysine – so it can bind to the plasminogen activator site instead of lysine and therefore block it from activating it in the first place.

There have been two good-quality, well-designed randomised controlled trials comparing the use of TXA 500mg daily with a placebo (and both groups using hydroquinone) over 8 and 12 weeks (300 patients total). Both studies showed a statistically significant improvement in melasma in the TXA group versus the placebo group. Importantly, no patients reported any adverse side effects from the TXA requiring the treatment to be stopped.[12]

> **The bottom line**: TXA can be an effective addition to your topical melasma treatment and the clinical trial evidence supports this. Talk to your doctor about whether it is right for you.

Cysteamine cream

Cysteamine cream has been known to be a depigmenting agent since 1966, when it was found to cause depigmentation via injection into the skin of black goldfish, and, later, as a topical treatment depigmenting the skin of black guinea pigs.

However, it is very unstable in a cream form and, when oxidised, produces an offensive odour. In 2010, new technology was used to reduce this odour, allowing it to be used as an ingredient in cosmetic skincare. But is it worth the hype and the price tag?

Two randomised placebo-controlled trials looking at the efficacy of 5 per cent cysteamine cream in the treatment of melasma found a significant improvement with the cysteamine cream versus a placebo.[13] However, I wouldn't recommend this cream over hydroquinone for several reasons, including cost, efficacy, ease of use and personalisation, not to mention decades'-worth of data supporting the safety and efficacy of hydroquinone.

It is interesting that the company that makes the cream has a disclaimer on their website stating that this product 'is not intended to . . . diagnose, treat, cure or prevent any disease or condition'. This, of course, contradicts how it is being marketed – as a treatment for melasma and pigmentation (or pigment 'correction').

PART 5

How to Tackle Common Aesthetic Concerns

No one watches the disfigurements, discolorations and deteriorations of ageing skin without anxiety and distress. We see our mortality in the skin's decadence. The psychological impacts are enormous.

Dr Arthur Balin and Dr Albert Kligman in
Aging and the Skin[1]

A good number of patients come to see me, not because they have a specific skin disease, but because they want to know how to either reverse some of the effects ageing and sun exposure have had on their skin or they want to prevent any from actually happening. I refer to these generally as 'cosmetic' concerns, though there is a strong overlap here with medical problems, like the deleterious effects of sun exposure causing pre-cancerous skin lesions or abnormal pigmentation like melasma. In this section, I am going to describe some of the most common cosmetic concerns I see in my clinic and what the most evidence-based treatments are (and what you should avoid!).

16

Fine Lines and Wrinkles

Wrinkles are visible creases or folds in the skin. Fine wrinkles are less than 1mm in width and depth, while coarse wrinkles are more than 1mm in width and depth. Though wrinkles can occur all over the face, the main areas of concern for most people are the forehead, which is the frontalis muscle, the crow's feet area around the eyes, which is the orbicularis oculi muscle, and the glabella complex (the 'elevenses') between the eyebrows, which is made up of the corrugators and the procerus muscles. Wrinkling is more common in white or fair-skinned people and the two biggest causes of wrinkles (apart from natural ageing) are sun exposure and smoking.[1]

A systematic review investigated all the possible treatments available for wrinkles.[2] After analysing 33 studies, they found the following: there is not enough evidence to suggest that chemical peels (both alpha and beta hydroxy peels), CO_2 laser, dermabrasion or variable pulsed erbium:YAG laser are effective at improving wrinkles. The topical retinoids tazarotene and tretinoin both had a positive effect on fine lines only, but both cause some skin irritation like redness and peeling.

We've already seen that the only FDA-approved topical treatment to improve the appearance of fine wrinkles is retinoic acid (tretinoin – see page 123). There have been at least 13 well-performed randomised controlled trials comparing tretinoin with a vehicle cream (the same cream base as the tretinoin cream, just without the tretinoin in it) in the treatment of wrinkles. The findings are that the daily application of tretin-oin cream at a concentration of 0.02 per cent or above may be more effective than the vehicle-only cream at improving wrin-kles after 16–48 weeks of continuous use in people with mild to severe photodamage. However, using a concentration less than 0.02 per cent may be no more effective than the vehicle cream at improving wrinkles.[3]

BOTULINUM TOXIN

The only intervention that was found to be consistently effective at improving wrinkles was the injection of botulinum toxin (also referred to generally as 'neurotoxin' or by the brand names such as 'Botox', 'Dysport' or 'Xeomin') with an effect that lasts up to 120 days (3 months) post-treatment. Side effects were mild and included headache and bruising at the injection sites immediately post-treatment. A one-sided drooping of the upper eyelid was noted in 25 (9 per cent) of subjects and this resolved on its own within 40 days of the treatment.[4] Botulinum toxin is now con-sidered the gold-standard treatment for dynamic facial wrinkles.

Botulinum toxin is a neurotoxin produced by the bacterium *Clostridium botulinum*. There are seven distinct types (named A to G) produced by different strains of the bacteria, but only the A and B types are available as drugs. In aesthetic medicine the A type is used predominantly, which is why you may see it being referred to as 'botulinum toxin type A'.

All the muscles in your body are controlled by nerves; this includes the muscles of your face. The nerves reach the muscles and, to tell the muscle to move, the nerves send a chemical signal called acetylcholine (ACH), which is a small protein molecule called a 'neurotransmitter' that is released from the nerve ending and travels across the small space between the nerve ending and the muscle to activate a receptor on the target muscle. When the receptor is activated, a cascade of events occurs within the mus-cle cell to tell it to move. Botulinum toxin blocks the release of

ACH from the end of the nerve at the space where the nerve endings touch the muscle (the neuromuscular junction).

Botulinum toxin has been used in medicine for various therapeutic reasons for over 30 years and in the cosmetic arena for over 25 years, with an impressive record of both safety and efficacy when used appropriately by well-trained and experienced injectors. Botulinum toxin was approved to treat wrinkles in 2002, but was first reported to reduce the appearance of facial wrinkles in 1990.[5]

SKINTELLIGENT TIP:

You won't be poisoned by your wrinkle injections

Botulinum toxin is 7 million times more toxic than cobra venom and a mere pint of it could kill every single human being on the planet. The name comes from the word 'botulism', which is a rare but serious illness in which the toxin is ingested from poorly sanitised tinned or processed food manufacturing. It attacks the body's nerves and causes difficulty with breathing, muscle paralysis and sometimes death. It was first reported back in the 1700s but is not commonly seen now due to strict food hygiene laws.

However, you won't get botulism from your wrinkle injections because the toxin is diluted and the dose used is tiny. It is super important to remember that (as with most things) the dose makes the poison.

Making sure your toxin is injected correctly

There is a pervading myth that injecting botulinum toxin for wrinkles is 'easy'. Yes, it is indeed easy to inject, but it is not easy to inject *correctly*. I can spot badly done botulinum toxin from a mile away and I often must 'correct' it when patients come to see me, having had injections elsewhere.

The biggest mistake I see on a regular basis is that there is too much movement in the forehead muscle above the outside or 'lateral wing' of the eyebrow (what people refer to as a 'Spock' brow after Dr Spock from *Star Trek*). This happens because botulinum toxin is injected into the middle third of the forehead to 'relax' that part of the muscle, but the patient has asked for an eyebrow 'lift' or the injector has promised a 'lift' and therefore does not inject into the lateral sides of the muscle. This results in the frontalis muscle on either side of the forehead being overactive and creating unnatural-looking wrinkles above the outside third of each eyebrow (the 'wings') every time the patient moves their forehead up. A little injection mid-way up the forehead on each side will immediately correct this and stop those funny-looking wrinkles from forming. You want a smooth forehead all across, not just in the middle!

It's important to remember that the effects of botulinum toxin are not immediate; the maximum effect can be seen after about

FACIAL MUSCLES THAT ARE THE TARGET FOR BOTULINUM TOXIN INJECTIONS

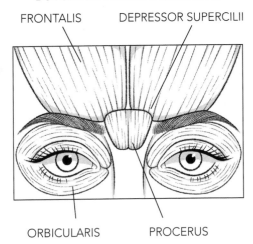

FRONTALIS   DEPRESSOR SUPERCILII

ORBICULARIS   PROCERUS

2 weeks and the duration is usually between 90 and 120 days, depending on the strength of the muscles treated and the dosages used. The 'paralysing' effect slowly wears off as the affected nerves grow new nerve terminals to restore the impaired signal transmission, and the nerve ending directly affected by the botulinum toxin will also regenerate its function. It is also important to note that there is no 'antidote' for botulinum toxin, meaning the effect cannot be reversed immediately. If you don't like the way it looks, the only thing you can do is wait for it to wear off.

There are several different botulinum toxin A products available on the market. Though some people claim one brand is different from or better than another, they are virtually all identical. The main difference is usually in the way it is dosed. Your injector will be familiar with whichever brand they use so will be able to dose it correctly.

If you have a lot of upper eyelid skin laxity or a 'hooded' upper lid, relaxing your forehead muscle may give you a heavy feeling in your eyelids or lower forehead. This is because if you have hooded upper lids you will tend to overuse your forehead muscle to allow your eyes to be more open, lifting the heavy eyelid; in other words, you may have 'hypertonicity' of your frontalis muscle so you can see better. If botulinum toxin is used to 'take away' your ability to raise your eyelids using your forehead muscle, you will invariably complain of a heavy brow and have difficulty, for example, opening your eyes wide enough to apply mascara. In this situation, I advise against botulinum toxin and suggest corrective surgery for the drooping or lax upper eyelid.

THE MOST COMMON QUESTIONS I GET ASKED ABOUT BOTULINUM TOXIN

Can botulinum toxin injections 'lift'?

The biggest misconception about botulinum toxin is that it can somehow create a 'lifting' effect of the eyelid or the eyebrows.

This is just not true. Botulinum toxin by its very nature relaxes muscles so they don't move when you want them to (some people call this 'paralysis'). A very misleading study was published in 2020 with the title 'Lifting effect of onabotulinumtoxin A in patients treated for glabellar and crow's feet rhytids'.[6] The researchers injected the glabella and crow's feet with botulinum toxin and observed an elevation of the entire eyebrow and upper eyelid post-treatment. It is important to remember that both the muscles targeted – the glabellar complex and the orbicularis oculi muscles (the ones that encircle the eye and allow you to squeeze your eyes shut) – are depressor muscles; they pull the eyelid and eyebrow down. As we age, these depressor muscles become stronger than the elevating frontalis muscle of the forehead and this can lead to the eyebrows and eyelids looking like they are sitting lower on the face than they were previously or a sad or tired appearance of the eye area.

If botulinum toxin is injected into these muscles, they relax and are no longer able to function as depressors, and the frontalis muscle of the forehead can then 'take over', giving a slight pull to the eyebrow and eyelid. Hence, a 'lift'. In the study, standard injections were done into the corrugator muscle and the procerus muscles of the glabellar complex and the crow's feet area. The forehead was not treated. Hence, a 'lift' occurred. But remember this isn't anything magical due to the botulinum toxin itself; it is the result of opposing muscle groups no longer opposing each other. The results themselves were tiny, with resting eyebrow height increasing by about 1.5mm on each side. That would be barely noticeable in real life. It is studies like this that are confusing and deceptive for patients who then seek out treatments with the hope of achieving a dramatic lift to their eyebrows, which can't really happen.

SKINTELLIGENT FACT:

Botulinum toxin immunity

'Neutralising antibodies' are small protein molecules that bind to the botulinum toxin when it is injected and therefore stop it from binding to the nerve ending. However, studies show that it is very rare for this to happen and for someone to become immune to botulinum toxin, and it is probably not relevant in the field of aesthetics.[7]

Does botulinum toxin prevent wrinkles from forming?

Skin wrinkles are created by the repeated use of muscles of the face. It is logical to therefore assume that if you stop using the muscles completely, the skin fold will no longer be made and you therefore smooth out the wrinkles present and, by no longer using the muscle and 'folding' the skin, you prevent wrinkles from forming.

Though there are no controlled long-term studies, one study found that botulinum toxin injections most likely prevent wrinkles.[8] However, you need to be consistent with it for years to really benefit. And that is a financial investment.

There is also evidence that regular, repeated treatments provide aesthetic benefits beyond just paralysis of the muscle. Although the exact mechanism is not known, there are some clinical studies and case reports that show that long-term use of botulinum toxin not only prevents formation of new wrinkles but also leads to progressive improvements in skin quality and improves the appearance of long-standing static wrinkles. Some studies even show that the time interval between sessions can become longer with consistent use without losing aesthetic benefits. That means you would need fewer injections (and to spend less money) while still getting the benefit of the treatment over time.[9]

The bottom line: Be regular and consistent with botulinum toxin injections to reap the long-term benefits. Of all the minimally invasive treatments available, botulinum toxin has by far the greatest efficacy, with the strongest scientific evidence base as well as a low level of risk and side effects, making it probably the best 'anti-ageing' treatment available right now.

SKINTELLIGENT TIP:

Bolutinum toxin injections may improve forehead acne

Interestingly, there is a relationship between sweating, oiliness and keratinisation (the accumulation of dead skin cells in the hair follicle). Though all these things are independent of each other, they seem to be unified in that if you get oilier and more keratinisation and perhaps more sweating, you end up with more acne. This may be one reason patients find that their forehead acne improves when they get botulinum toxin injections into the forehead for wrinkles. People often say it is because the neurotoxin reduces oil secretion, but we know that is not the case. However, it does affect the eccrine glands by blocking the nerve that controls the function of the sweat gland (neurotoxin blocks the release of ACH, which is the neurotransmitter that gives the signal to activate the sweat gland to produce sweat). Hence, less forehead sweat means less oiliness.

17

Dark Under-Eye Circles

I n the scientific literature, dark under-eye circles are referred to as 'cutaneous idiopathic hyperchromia of the orbital region' (CIHOR).[1] But to people who suffer from them, they're just annoying: those dark circles that never go away, no matter how much sleep you get or how many different vitamin C or caffeine-infused lotions and potions you religiously apply to the area.

Is it possible to get rid of them, for good? Well, to be totally honest, no, you can't. But let me explain why and what you can do to help improve the appearance of your under-eye area before you stop reading and throw this book in the bin.

WHAT CAUSES UNDER-EYE CIRCLES?

The first step to finding a solution is to understand the problem. One way to diagnose what is happening in skin is to take a piece of the skin and look at it under a microscope – called a skin biopsy. This can help to identify abnormalities in 'diseased' skin that aren't present in normal skin. And that's exactly what a group of researchers did to investigate what is going on in the skin of people with dark under-eye circles: they found an increase in melanin (what gives your skin colour – the pigment), dilation or widening of the blood vessels in the upper dermis of the skin and a decrease in blood oxygen levels (so poor circulation), compared to the normal skin behind the patients' ears.[2] The amount of melanin, dilation of vessels and low oxygen saturation levels increased the darker the circles were.

So, why does this happen? No one really knows, but there is a lot of research trying to figure this out because it is such a common and annoying problem. There is a good amount of evidence that the development of dark under-eye circles is hereditary, especially if you have a female relative (mother or grandmother) who has the same problem. Interestingly, studies have also found an association between asthma and the development of dark under-eye circles, though the reason why this connection exists is unclear.[3] It might be because, if you have asthma, you are more likely to be 'atopic', meaning you have allergies in general or this runs in your family. Atopy is known to result in inflammation around the eyes and poor circulation in the area as well, which is probably a big factor in causing the problem. Chronic inflammation around the eyes for whatever reason will result in a disruption of the pigment-producing cells in the skin and, in turn, cause more pigment to be deposited in the skin in that area. There is no relationship between hay fever, eczema, alcohol use or having acne and dark under-eye circles.[4]

In addition, there is no evidence that sleep deprivation is linked to dark under-eye circles.[5] You might have noticed this yourself – no matter how much rest you get, you still have the under-eye darkness. There seems to be a cultural bias associating dark circles or their absence with general well-being or lack of sleep. For example, in Japanese, there are several words describing dark under-eye circles, which can also refer to exhaustion or sickness! But there is little evidence that this is actually true.

One big thing that is often forgotten about is your anatomy – the way your orbital bones 'sit' and how much fat you have on your face.[6] As you age, you lose the youthful fat around your eyes, and the bones around your eyes – your orbital bones – can become more prominent. This causes problems because it can cause shadows to develop under your eyes, which are then seen as the dreaded 'dark circles'. There is also a ligament that separates the lower under-eye area from your cheek – referred to as the 'tear trough' ligament. This is the anatomical basis for the crevice between the mid-cheek and lower eyelid, near the nose or corner of the eye, that is more pronounced in some than in others.

HOW TO REDUCE THE APPEARANCE OF DARK CIRCLES

One really interesting way to correct this more pronounced depression is through the very careful placement of a hyaluronic acid filler into the under-eye area (the tear trough). When done well, this can slightly plump up the crevice, smoothening the 'step' between the lower lid and the mid-cheek and improving the appearance of under-eye dark circles. However, the majority of people don't have the right type of tear trough 'deformity' that can be corrected with filler (only one out of every ten of my patients is suitable for tear trough filler), though those who do see an immediate improvement with very little filler. If you want to try this and discuss other surgical options, please make sure you find a qualified and experienced plastic surgeon, oculoplastic surgeon or dermatologist to guide you and perform the procedure, as well as explaining to you the rare but serious complications that can occur if this procedure is done incorrectly.

Short-term changes in the appearance of your under-eye circles can also be due to dehydration, though this plays only a minor role. Your body is really good at regulating its fluid status (hydration levels) if you are otherwise well, but this might be one reason to keep your water intake up during the day; the general recommendation is to drink 6–8 cups or glasses of fluid a day and one way for you to monitor your hydration levels is the colour of your wee: a light yellow colour is a good indicator that you are well-hydrated.[7]

Visually, studies have shown that the severity of dark under-eye circles is directly related to the contrast between the darkened under-eye skin and the surrounding cheek skin. This is pretty obvious, but has been confirmed by research.[8] So trying to 'match' your under-eye skin with your cheek skin via make-up is a good step forward in at least temporarily correcting the problem.

Yes, dark under-eye circles are a cosmetic nuisance and there is no way to get rid of them permanently. Whether you have them because your mother does or because you have an underlying predisposition to allergies or asthma, these factors are not something that you can change. From my clinical experience, the most common reason for dark under-eye circles is that they are hereditary. The majority of these patients have lower eyelids that are relatively translucent, allowing for the underlying vasculature (blood vessels) to be seen and imparting a deep purple hue to the skin under the eyes. If you stretch the skin under the eye of these patients, the violaceous or purple hue should deepen and this confirms a vascular cause. This type of dark under-eye circle is not always amenable to correction with tear trough filler because the tear trough is not always pronounced – but, if it is, that can be corrected to help improve the entire lower eyelid appearance.

I also recommend using a topical retinoid, which, over time, should increase the collagen in the dermis to further help 'plump' the skin and bring about some subtle improvement. Just be cautious when applying retinoids too close to the lower lash line because it can be quite irritating to the eyes if it gets in them and it can also temporarily dry the skin of the lower eyelid, especially at the beginning of treatment. Definitely use Vaseline as your eye cream to help reduce any dryness!

18

Unwanted or Excess Facial Hair

There are myriad ways to remove hair from the face – shaving, plucking, epilation (which is electronic plucking), creams (chemical depilation), waxing, threading ... but these are all temporary, and many people want something permanent. But before we explore hair removal options, let me emphasise that **it is *normal* and *natural* to have hair on your face.** There are 730 follicles per cm² on the face alone – that's a lot of hair![1]

There are two types of hair on your face:

1. Terminal hairs: the darker, thicker hairs.
2. Vellus hairs: the finer, lighter hairs that cover most of your face and body.

Women develop terminal hairs on their face almost exclusively due to hormonal changes or disruption, where androgens are the culprit. (Androgens are the hormones responsible primarily for male growth and development and women have small amounts as well.) This can happen mainly at three times in your life: when you go through puberty, in your teens and early twenties due to polycystic ovary syndrome (PCOS) and then again in your forties or fifties as part of perimenopause or menopause. The pattern of hair development can be similar, but it tends to be more widespread and thicker in patients with PCOS and more localised to the chin and upper lip area in perimenopausal women. The medical term for this is 'hirsutism', which means 'male pattern' hair growth on areas where women would normal not get hair growth (the side-burns, chin and upper lip) and affects up to 10 per cent of women globally.[2]

PCOS is a condition characterised by excess androgen hormones in women, and results in these patients having menstrual irregularities, hirsutism, acne vulgaris and female pattern hair loss.[3] If you feel you have this condition, see your GP or healthcare professional to confirm the diagnosis and explore the most appropriate management plan for you. Though this is not my area of expertise, the one thing I have observed through clinical practice is the impact of diet on the symptoms of PCOS. Of all the conditions I see in dermatology, the only one (aside from medically-diagnosed food allergies like coeliac disease) that responds to a dietary change is PCOS. I often advise my patients to consider a low-sugar, low-refined-carbohydrate diet as part of their management plan. If you think this might work for you, I strongly advise you to speak to your doctor or a qualified dietician.

SKINTELLIGENT FACT:

Idiopathic hirsutism

'Idiopathic hirsutism' is the term used to describe male pattern hair growth in women without an underlying cause (idiopathic means it comes on spontaneously, without an underlying cause). Women often believe or are told that they have a 'hormonal imbalance' causing their excess hair growth. Though this may be true, like in PCOS or during menopause, it is not something that is generally measurable because the problem isn't that androgens are 'too high', but that the hair follicle is more sensitive to androgens. That's why if you were to check your blood androgen levels, they would almost certainly be normal.

Treatment of hirsutism if related to androgens like in PCOS requires a two-pronged approach: reducing the androgen 'drive' to the hair follicle and getting rid of the actual hair that is present.[4] Reduction of the androgen drive is important because, once the terminal hair is present, the only way to remove it is through destruction of the hair or hair follicle. There are several tablet treatments available to help reduce the androgen drive:

- Metformin: works to reduce the levels of circulating insulin in the body, which then decreases free androgen concentrations, thus improving hirsutism.
- Cyproterone acetate: a progestogen that has anti-androgen effects. It is often combined with oestrogen in a combined contraceptive pill.
- Flutamide: another anti-androgen.
- Spironolactone: a potassium-sparing diuretic with some anti-androgen activity.
- Finasteride: works by inhibiting the enzyme 5-alpha-reductase, which converts testosterone to the active form dihydrotestosterone. This is not specifically licensed for the treatment of hirsutism and should not be used by women of childbearing age.

As you can see, there are several options available to you so definitely speak to your doctor.

If you think you have hirsutism, it is vital that you identify the cause of it and treat any androgen excess medically. If you don't and you get hair removal treatments, you will almost certainly continue to see conversion of vellus to terminal hairs in the treated areas, which you may view as the treatment having failed.

Even if you only have idiopathic hirsutism (normal androgen levels, but you are hypersensitive to androgens – see box above), you may still have some vellus to terminal hair conversion in androgen-dependent areas like the upper lip and chin. Seeking medical advice in conjunction with your choice of hair removal treatment is vital to ensuring a successful long-term resolution.

HAIR REMOVAL

If your hair is darker or more visible, thicker, coarser or just in very specific areas like your upper lip or chin (or you just don't like it), it makes absolute sense to want to get rid of it, permanently. There are two types of hair removal that can offer longer-lasting results: laser/intense pulsed light and electrolysis.

Lasers and intense pulsed light

Lasers and intense pulsed light (IPL) work by targeting the melanin pigment in unwanted hair. Because these systems use only a specific wavelength of light, the damage they create is only to the hair follicles, so surrounding structures, like the skin itself, remain undamaged. When it comes to laser hair removal, if you have lots of dark, thick hair and you are pale, probably the best hair removal laser for you is going to be an Alexandrite laser (755nm) or a diode (810nm). If you have lots of dark, thick hair and you have darker or more olive skin, then an Nd:YAG (1064nm) laser is the best one for you. But lasers aren't my preferred method for facial hair removal because it's not permanent and can stimulate more hair growth, a phenomenon referred to as 'paradoxical hypertrichosis'.

Paradoxical hypertrichosis is an uncommon, poorly understood negative effect associated with laser or IPL treatment for hair removal.[5] It tends to occur as new dark hair appearing in the area of skin outside the boundaries of the area actually treated with the laser. While exactly why this occurs is not known, one of the most probable explanations is that it is due to treatment with 'suboptimal fluencies' (too low power), which leads to conversion of vellus hairs to terminal hairs. It was first described in 2002 and a systematic review published in 2021 found that 4 per cent of patients experienced paradoxical hypertrichosis, but the occurrence rate varied massively between studies – from 0 to 62 per cent![6] It does mostly occur in facial hair removal though and is extremely rare in non-facial areas (a low prevalence of only 0.08 per cent). This may be because there are a lot more vellus hairs on the face than any other part of the body and the problem is the conversion of vellus to terminal hairs. There may be an association with skin colour, as paradoxical hypertrichosis seems to occur more frequently in those with Fitzpatrick skin types III–IV, compared with lighter skin types I–II (see page 34). It also only seems to occur after at least three treatment sessions and even as late as six months after the last (eighth) session. This fits with the idea that hair induction (stimulation of new hair growth) is a slow process and requires time to develop.

So how do you fix it if this happens to you? It is probably best to continue laser treatment and treat those affected areas as well, as they appear to respond to laser treatment. The type of laser or IPL device you have does not seem to impact whether you will experience paradoxical hypertrichosis.

SKINTELLIGENT TIP:

Snip hair between laser or IPL treatments

Something I get asked quite often by patients is whether it's best to snip or shave facial hair between laser or IPL treatments. This has actually been studied on patients receiving laser hair removal for chin hair.

> The conclusion was that it's probably better to use scissors to snip your hair between treatments if you want to optimise long-term outcome.[7] Don't pluck, wax or thread hairs while undergoing treatment.

A key with laser hair removal is that for the FDA to approve a laser for hair removal, the laser (or any hair removal device) must have clinical trial evidence showing a sustained reduction in hair growth for a three-month period only. Interestingly, the first laser approved by the FDA for hair removal was only in 1995. None of the lasers discussed here have been proven to permanently destroy hair – they just slow regrowth.

Hair grows through three phases:

1. The anagen phase: the active growth phase of the hair cycle – lasts 2–6 years on the scalp, 1–2 months for the eyebrow and 2–5 months for the upper lip. In people with hormone- or age-related hair loss, the length of the anagen phase decreases dramatically.
2. The catagen phase: this is only two weeks long and is when the hair is shed.
3. The telogen phase: the 'resting' phase of the hair cycle, when the hair does not grow and, again, the length of this phase changes according to body site (3–4 months on the scalp and the eyebrows, 1.5 months on the upper lip).

Only anagen hairs are sensitive to the effects of injury (such as by laser). When the hair follicle is injured, this can cause a prolonged delay to regrowth because injury can trigger a telogen-to-anagen switch of all the hairs in the treated area. This causes all the hairs to start growing at the same time after a certain amount of time not growing, synchronising the hair cycle, meaning that you don't see regrowth for quite some time post-treatment.[8] This means that laser hair removal is not permanent – you will require ongoing 'top-up' treatments to keep your face (and body) hair-free in the long run.

What if you have darker skin?

Research has shown that patients with more pigmented skin (Fitzpatrick skin types III–VI) are prone to experiencing more side effects from laser treatments.[9] A review of the literature shows that, in terms of hair reduction, the long-pulsed Nd:YAG laser and the diode laser were similar to IPL, while the Alexandrite laser was found to be superior to IPL. However, when it came to causing post-inflammatory hyperpigmentation (PIH), the long-pulsed Nd:YAG was less likely to cause this side effect when compared to IPL, and the Alexandrite and diode caused similar amounts of PIH compared to IPL. The lasers did cause more pain generally than IPL. Overall, the treatment outcomes for patients of darker skin were broadly similar across all modalities, though the trend did favour greater hair reduction with the lasers rather than IPL.

Electrolysis

The gold standard for facial hair removal is electrolysis. I know what you are thinking – 'That's so old-fashioned! Do people still do that?'. Well, call me old-fashioned, but electrolysis is still the only permanent method of hair removal. Yes, it can be painful (but so is laser hair removal) and it is fairly time-consuming, but when you zap the hair at the right part of the hair cycle, it is a permanent destruction of the hair. If you can find a good, convenient electrolysis technician, go for that – you will be happy you did in the long run. I usually suggest starting with weekly treatments and then spacing them out depending on your regrowth. Your technician should give you a treatment plan with a rough idea of how many hours of treatment you will require to achieve clearance of your hair. But remember, just like laser, you can't pluck, wax or thread between treatments.

Electrolysis has been around since 1875. What exact part of the hair follicle needs to be destroyed to achieve destruction of the hair completely is still up for debate – it is probably the bottom or lower half (called the dermal papilla), but there is some evidence to suggest that the hair can regenerate from the upper portions of the hair follicle as well, even if the bottom – where the regenerating cells live – has been destroyed. Nevertheless, it is still widely believed that the dermal papillae need to be destroyed for permanent hair removal to occur and we have evidence that electrolysis does indeed achieve that.[10]

Scarring does not generally occur with proper electrolysis technique, and it can be done on any skin type and on any hair type (vellus, terminal, of any colour, thickness) and on any part of the body. It involves the insertion of a very fine needle directly into the hair follicle, and either a direct or alternating electric current is applied to the hair.[11] When the needle is inserted correctly and the hair is treated sufficiently, it should be gently lifted out of the follicle with fine tweezers. If you feel a 'pluck' then the treatment has not been done properly. The results are extremely technician-dependent, so finding someone who has experience and is well-trained in electrolysis is absolutely essential and also, in some parts of the world, a real challenge.

Electrolysis can leave you with redness and swelling around the treated hair follicles, but this is temporary. It is a treatment that is safe on tanned skin as well as people using topical treatments like retinoic acid and on oral isotretinoin. Electrolysis has never been shown to stimulate skin problems or conditions such as vitiligo, rosacea or acne.

Other things to consider

Eflornithine cream

Eflornithine cream, known by its brand name Vaniqa, is the first and only prescription treatment approved by the MHRA and FDA for the reduction of unwanted facial hair in women. It works by irreversibly inhibiting an enzyme called ornithine decarboxylase, which is necessary for hair growth. With continued daily use, it can slow down the growth of unwanted facial hair by up to 60 per cent, but this occurs gradually over 4–8 weeks or longer. The only adverse reaction is minor skin irritation.[12] However, it does not permanently stop hair growth, so it needs to be used in conjunction with other hair removal techniques. Hair growth returns to pretreatment levels within eight weeks of stopping the cream.[13] Vaniqa is only available on prescription, so if this is something you want to try, speak to your doctor.

Dermaplaning

Dermaplaning is the use of a sharp blade to remove the top layers of the skin (the stratum corneum) along with the hair from your face with the aim of making the skin surface look smoother and supposedly to 'remove' fine lines and deep acne scarring. Basically, it's shaving your face and will have zero impact on fine lines and deep acne scarring. But it will indeed remove the top layer of the stratum corneum and, of course, all the hair on your face (mainly the 'peach fuzz').

Dermaplaning was first reported in the scientific literature back in the 1970s as a treatment for various skin problems including acne vulgaris. Back in the day, they used either a scalpel blade or an automatic machine like the ones used now to take skin for split-thickness skin grafts. This procedure was generally done by plastic surgeons.

Dermaplaning is a trendy 'beauty treatment' now – you can get it done by a beautician as part of a facial or you can purchase specific razors so you can do this 'in the comfort of your own home', with gadgets ranging in price from just under £200 to a couple of quid for a standard plastic-handled razor from your local supermarket.

There is no published scientific literature about the use of dermaplaning and its effects on the skin – positive or negative. The only time I have ever done anything close to dermaplaning is when I treated rhinophyma (excess skin growth on the noses of men with long-standing rosacea) with an infrared device during my surgical fellowship. We used this device to basically shave off the overgrowth of skin on the noses of men with rhinophyma, to give them back a more 'normal-looking' nose.

Aside from that, I don't know of any true reason for dermaplaning today. We don't need to do it for acne because we have much safer, less damaging treatments that can clear acne. The very top layers of skin (the stratum corneum) are there for a reason and removing them with a sharp blade is totally unnecessary in my opinion. It may temporarily make your skin feel softer or smoother because you have removed any dry, slightly rough skin and also the vellus (fine) hair on your face, but it is not a true treatment for anything.

The absolute most common concern all women have with shaving their face is: will the hair grow back thicker? The scientific evidence shows that shaving does not change the thickness or growth rate of human hair.[14] I know you may find this hard to believe if you have personally experienced increased hair growth after shaving yourself, and I do not discredit what you have experienced, but let me explain the science. The actively growing part of the hair is the root, and this is located in the deep dermis. Any procedure that is directed only at the fully keratinised, metabolically inactive hair shaft above the skin surface theoretically should not influence hair growth. However, the studies that this is based on were performed on the legs and chests of men and not on the faces of women. I cannot find any studies performed on the faces of women. For shaving to stimulate thicker, darker hair to grow in place of the shaved vellus hair, the vellus hair would need to convert into terminal hair via the root. This seems to be possible with regards to the use of laser or lights (as described on page 249), but how or why this would happen in response to shaving is not clear. It is possible that shaving causes the tip of the hair to have a rough texture compared with the softer, tapered tip of uncut hair and this may give the impression of thickening. Though I can't provide an evidence base for this statement, I will advise you not to shave your facial hair as it appears in some patients to grow back thicker and darker over time.

On the other hand, there is a notion out there that if you shave your eyebrows, they won't grow back. This isn't true – they will – it's been studied![15]

EYELASH AND EYEBROW HYPOTRICHOSIS (THIN/SHORT EYELASHES)

I have yet to meet a woman who does not covet beautiful, long, thick eyelashes. They frame the eyes, making them look wider and brighter. .The entire mascara industry is based on the idea that long, fabulous eyelashes are within everyone's reach.

But before you go out to buy another tube of mascara or invest in lash extensions, there is one product on the market that really does the trick. It's called bimatoprost and it's a prescription eye drop treatment used for glaucoma.

I know what you are thinking – is this for real? Yes, it is. Glaucoma is a serious medical condition that affects older people and causes increased pressure in the eye. Doctors noticed a while ago that patients treated with bimatoprost eye drops, which lower the pressure in the eye, also developed long eyelashes. Allergan, the company that makes Botox, picked up on this and found that if you apply bimatoprost like eyeliner to the upper lash line only, it will have the same effect. And they have now started selling this product as a prescription-only medicine under the brand name Latisse.

Does it work? Absolutely! I have been using it for years to grow my short little eyelashes into the long wispy lashes they are now. Mind you, it doesn't make your lashes thicker, just longer. It does this by stopping the hair cycle right before the hair is meant to shed (it prolongs the anagen phase and does not allow the hair to enter telogen, so it continues to grow beyond what it is genetically programmed to do). Eventually you do shed the hair, but not before it gets noticeably longer.

There are side effects though. It can change your eye pressure, so it's best to get this checked before starting treatment and every six months during the treatment. There is also a very small risk that it can darken light blue or green eyes and cause darkening of the skin around the eyelashes.[16] Although darkened eyelids might fade when the medication is stopped, any changes in iris colour are likely to be permanent.[17]

POTENTIAL SIDE EFFECTS OF LATISSE

- redness of the thin tissue over the white part of the eye (conjunctiva)
- itchy, red eyes – this is the most common side effect and is seen in 4 per cent of people in clinical trials
- dry eyes
- darkened eyelids
- darkened brown pigmentation in the coloured part of the eye (iris) – this takes months to years to become apparent
- hair growth around the eyes if the medication regularly runs or drips off the eyelids

Another side effect is known as periorbital fat atrophy – a hollowed-out appearance of the eyelids. This fat atrophy is permanent and can be severe. However, this side effect is rare.[18]

The recommended use of bimatoprost for eyelash growth is once daily at night to the upper lash line and full results should be apparent 3–4 months into treatment – so stick with it and don't expect results too quickly. And remember, to maintain the effect on your eyelashes you must continue to use it. If and when you stop it, your eyelashes will return to their original appearance.[19]

This is a prescription medication, so you need to speak to your doctor to see if it is right for you.

19

Skin 'Rejuvenation'

S kin rejuvenation generally refers to the overall improvement of the appearance of the skin – for it to be smoother, tighter and softer, with fewer fine lines and wrinkles. The focus of skin rejuvenation treatments is usually the dermis – at least that's what Big Skincare is trying to make you believe! In Part 1 we learnt all about collagen in the dermis – how it's made, what it does and how its structure in the dermis changes with age (see pages 28 and 52). What, if anything, can be done to improve the structure and function of the dermis, to 'rejuvenate' the skin?

There are many, many 'treatments' on the market that are meant to tighten and 'lift' sagging skin, though few have had any decent scientific evaluation of their efficacy. This is an incredibly confusing area of 'aesthetic' medicine, to say the least. If we take a critical, evidence-based approach, the best way to make sense of all the available treatments is to put them into five categories:

1. Systemic treatments: tablets or capsules you swallow.
2. Topical treatments: products you apply to the skin surface, like creams.
3. Injectable treatments: products that are injected into the skin with a needle.
4. Heat-, light- or 'energy'-based treatments: applied to the skin surface.

5. Mechanical treatments: suspending skin with sutures or 'threads' or needling the skin.

Virtually all treatments in the arena of skin rejuvenation are aiming to do one thing: stimulate new collagen (and, to some extent, elastin) production in the skin, which could theoretically lead to tightening, smoothening and lifting of the skin. This is called 'neocollagenesis' (see page 54). We know that this is a very slow process. The aim of stimulating new collagen production is to shift the balance from breakdown of collagen due to ageing in favour of the production of new collagen, while also ensuring that the new collagen created is not fragmented or disordered. Even if the new collagen formed is primarily fibrotic type III collagen, that may still benefit the appearance of skin by theoretically making the dermis more firm or 'rigid'.

SKINTELLIGENT TIP:

'Facials' are a total waste of time and money

Though relaxing and potentially enjoyable, from a skin benefit point of view, facials are totally pointless and potentially harmful for your skin in the long run. One study looked at 142 women (aged 17–63) for 12 weeks after getting a standard facial. What they found was quite shocking:[1]

- Thirty-three per cent developed an acneiform eruption 3–10 weeks after the facial, characterised by deep-seated nodules mainly on the cheeks along with closed comedones (basically – the facial gave them acne).

- Five per cent developed facial dermatitis 2–7 days after the facial and 4 of these patients were found to have patch test positive contact allergies to constituents of the products used in the facial.
- No objective benefits or improvement in facial skin were found.

Why did the facial cause acne in these patients? Thirty-seven patients with acneiform eruptions appearing on average 6.2 weeks post-facial were studied. Clinical and biopsy studies of these patients' skin showed that:[2]

- All had deep-seated nodules and scattered, closed comedones on the cheeks, with 18.9 per cent also having them on the forehead and 24.3 per cent on the chin.
- Patients who got regular facials (every 3–6 weeks) had persistent presence of these specific lesions (so they were there all the time).
- Biopsies of the nodules showed histology in keeping with the underlying cause for the acne being due to the massage of the skin, probably due to irritation or disruption of the structure of the pilosebaceous unit (as opposed to the idea that the creams used during the facial are 'comedogenic').

So, save your time and your money and skip the facial completely.

SYSTEMIC TREATMENTS

Though taking tablets to stimulate skin rejuvenation sounds fabulous, in reality there are very few things that can stimulate collagen production from the inside. The only two possibilities are hormone replacement therapy and oral isotretinoin.

Hormone replacement therapy (HRT)

Thirty per cent of skin collagen is lost within five years of menopause, and studies have demonstrated that taking oestrogen as HRT can stimulate new collagen formation.[3] Though HRT is a whole-body and therefore 'systemic' treatment, it is usually taken as a combination of a cream or a gel with a pill or a patch, depending on what you need specifically. Your GP, healthcare professional or menopause specialist doctor is the best person to discuss this with. It is important to remember that HRT is taken to tackle the symptoms of menopause (which can vary from person to person) and usually not specifically for skin.

Oral isotretinoin

Both topical tretinoin and oral isotretinoin are vitamin A derivatives (see Chapter 7). Topical tretinoin has a well-established evidence base for the improvement of fine lines of photoaged skin, but what about oral isotretinoin?

A very thorough review article searched the literature and found 6 studies with a total of 251 subjects relating to this question.[4] Four studies showed that oral isotretinoin seemed to improve photoaged skin, one showed no benefit and one showed no benefit in comparison to topical tretinoin. Unfortunately, these studies all suffer from major methodological problems, such as small sample sizes, lack of controls and non-blinded observers. The authors conclude that there is a lack of high-quality studies to determine if oral isotretinoin is an effective and safe alternative for the treatment of photoageing.

The bottom line: Stick with topical tretinoin as the most evidence-based treatment for photoaged skin.

TOPICAL TREATMENTS

We have already covered the gold-standard topical treatment for skin rejuvenation – topical retinoic acid, or tretinoin. Is there anything else that can possibly reverse the photodamage you may already have?

Strong experimental evidence shows that the skin can repair itself quite significantly, even within a few months, if UV exposure (sun exposure) is stopped.[5] What seems to happen in the dermis is that new collagen is made in the very top of the dermis, just below the epidermis, and this pushes the old, damaged elastin and collagen fibres downwards. The new collagen formed is normal, while the new elastic fibres are sparse and delicate. More experiments done in animals showed that, with the use of sunscreens, further damage can be prevented and even repair initiated, even with ongoing sun exposure. When the experimental animals were exposed to UV light with sunscreen protection, a repair zone of new subepidermal collagen was deposited in the upper levels of the dermis. In these studies, the sunscreens used were of an SPF6 and 15! But remember, these were animals, not humans. Obviously, a higher SPF (when used properly – see page 88) provides a greater degree of protection against photodamage.

The bottom line: Photoaged skin is not irreversibly damaged; if the UV exposure is continued, destruction and repair appear to go on simultaneously. The balance can be shifted towards repair if the UV insult is stopped, and the skin is protected with sunscreen.

INJECTABLE TREATMENTS ('FILLERS')

We usually think of fillers as a way to replace lost volume in the face. There are also fillers that are supposedly designed to improve the appearance of the skin over time by stimulating collagen production – neocollagenesis (see page 54). Fillers that stimulate neocollagenesis can be divided into 'inflammatory' fillers (those that stimulate inflammation and therefore a wound-healing response) and 'non-inflammatory' fillers. In both cases, new collagen creation occurs due to the stimulation of fibroblasts (the cells in the dermis that produce collagen). A key distinction is that 'inflammatory' fillers do not create immediate volume, while 'non-inflammatory' fillers can be used to create volume. The theory is that mechanical stress on the fibroblast caused by the injection of any filler will induce neocollagenesis by stimulation of fibroblasts, and maximum collagen is formed from the associated inflammatory reaction or when the filler being injected is in the form of microspheres.[6]

The most commonly used filler in the world today is cross-linked hyaluronic acid (HA – see page 151). It is a dissolving, temporary filler and, depending on the viscosity (thickness) of the filler used, it can be used to add volume to specific areas of the face or just be injected into the dermis without adding volume, to induce 'bioremodelling'. HA injected into the dermis can improve skin's appearance by stretching fibroblasts and stimulating collagen production. Studies have shown that, within one month of the injection of HA filler, collagen production substantially increases and remains high for at least three months post-injection.[7] Biopsies of the treated areas show that lots of fibroblasts congregate around the sites of the HA injections in the dermis. They appear to be stretched and elongated, and express high levels of type I procollagen (a precursor to collagen – see page 28). The HA possibly also acts as structural support in the dermis.

Poly-L-lactic acid (PLLA) is an inflammatory filler that is considered 'semi-permanent'. When injected, the PLLA micro-particles stimulate fibroblasts to produce more collagen fibres and cause a thicker dermis. Post-injection (every four weeks for three sessions), one study shows an over 33 per cent increase in type I collagen at six months post-treatment, with improvement lasting at least twenty-five months, if not several years. It is important to remember that the results are gradual, and it is not an immediate volume-enhancing filler.[8]

There are new fillers on the market that are being touted as 'biostimulators', which are non-inflammatory fillers. Calcium hydroxylapatite (CaHa) is a permanent, semi-solid filler com-posed of microspheres that can add immediate volume and has been shown to have a biostimulatory effect – it stimulates new collagen and elastin in the dermis via activation of fibroblasts – that appears to be sustained and present for at least 30 months post-injection.[9]

Polymethylmethacrylate (PMMA) is another microsphere, non-inflammatory filler and may continue to improve volume up to five years after injection by stimulating neocollagenesis. This is a permanent filler though and has a high risk of leaving lumps in the skin, so it is not used for treating lips or tear troughs (the space between the lower eyelid and the upper cheek, which can become more pronounced as we age due to volume loss – see page 243). It has been most studied for the treatment of atrophic acne scars.[10] Another new filler like this, based on the concept of microspheres, is polycaprolactone (PCL).[11]

Injectable hydrators

The idea of 'injecting' moisture into skin is not a new idea. It is well-recognised that HA in the dermis of the skin is partly responsible for skin 'plumpness' by holding water in the der-mis and it may also increase the production of collagen and other components of the dermis. As we age, the amount of HA in the dermis decreases. Because HA is a large molecular weight molecule (see page 116), it does not penetrate the skin when applied topically. Therefore, the idea of injecting it directly into the dermis to replenish and rejuvenate the skin was considered a logical next step.

One study showed improvement of cheek skin elasticity and skin roughness in nineteen female patients after a series of three sets of injections of HA spaced four weeks apart.[12] However, this study did not have a control group (which would use saline injections as a placebo), which is a major issue because it is possible that microneedling alone will induce inflammation and swelling in the skin, which will temporarily improve the appearance of fine lines and skin texture.

I have done a fairly extensive literature review a number of times over the past few years and I cannot find a vehicle-controlled study of these 'injectable hydrators'. The 'medical device' FDA approval for this specific product was gained in 2014 and the clinical study of efficacy looked at the use of it for lip augmentation and the correction of wrinkles around the lips only, and used a 'no-treatment' control – so not specifically as a skin 'hydrator'.

That being said, there is emerging evidence to suggest that cross-linked HA injected into the dermis can stimulate collagen production long-term. Though this isn't necessarily 'hydration', it may improve the overall appearance of skin.

ENERGY-BASED TREATMENTS

The market is currently saturated with various 'in-office' procedures or at-home devices to 'boost' the collagen in your dermis. Options include the use of different light sources (lasers, intense pulsed light (IPL) or LED), radiofrequency (fractional, mono or bipolar) and ultrasound (which is basically heat – the sound waves are absorbed and their energy is converted to heat), as well as various forms of microneedling.

All these methods claim to stimulate the production of collagen in the skin. The idea that somehow wounding or damaging the dermis will stimulate a repair mechanism, resulting in new collagen production and thus some skin tightening and 'rejuvenation', is, on the face of it, quite logical. After all, we know that if you damage the skin, it will repair itself (though usually not perfectly or exactly as it was prior to the damage being inflicted).

The idea here is that heat will denature (break apart) collagen. This happens somewhere between 65 and 70°C and is what initiates an inflammatory, wound-healing response in the dermis. However, it takes a lot of damage to stimulate a repair response of any visible or clinical significance. And any treatment that causes a lot of damage will necessitate a certain amount of 'downtime' (recovery) for the patient.

Though the CO_2 laser is still the gold standard to achieve true skin rejuvenation, the aesthetic industry is constantly trying to find an alternative that is just as effective with the absolute minimum required recovery afterwards. This has led to the introduction of alternative treatments like non-ablative laser resurfacing and other 'low-intensity' treatments, which generally provide minimal, if any, improvement to the skin. Basically, they just don't cause enough damage to the skin. Any improvement seen is short-term due to inflammation and swelling occurring in the dermis post-treatment.

'Non-surgical' facelifts

High-frequency ultrasound (HIFU, marketed under the brand name 'Ultherapy') is meant to 'heat' the facial tissue, denaturing the collagen, and then the collagen is meant to reform, making it 'stronger' and then you are meant to get skin tightening. Radiofrequency ('Thermage') also works by heating the tissue with electrical energy.

The issue is that a sagging face is not due to 'just' collagen loss in the dermis – so even if the treatment does stimulate new collagen, will it result in a 'facelift' type result? Perhaps temporarily, but definitely not permanently.

All the studies I have reviewed about these treatments that show improvement with these machines involve very carefully selected patients – younger women with mild tissue sagging only.[13] But even then, if results are seen, they are subtle and short-lived.

Considering how expensive, painful and time-consuming these 'non-surgical' options are, most women are probably better off saving their money and time for a proper surgical facelift.

SKINTELLIGENT TIP:

Using HIFU to achieve an eyebrow lift isn't worth the money

According to the FDA, you can get an eyebrow lift from HIFU – sort of. Ultherapy received FDA approval as a medical device in 2009 specifically for eyebrow lifting. This implies that it is safe and effective for its intended use. But how stringent is this process?

Medical devices are not the same as drugs and don't usually require the same type of clinical trial data to be approved (see page 113). Ultherapy is a class II device, which means it is deemed as 'moderate risk' and therefore the approval process is focused on registration, manufacturing and labelling, and does not require extensive pre-clinical or clinical data to establish efficacy. Some class II devices qualify for 'exempt' status, meaning that there is no need at all to prove safety or efficacy.

Ultherapy got approved as a medical device, but not because it does what it says it is going to do. The first clinical study done in live humans was published in 2010.[14] This was a trial to see if HIFU could give a brow lift in 36 subjects. The methods used to complete this uncontrolled study are fairly dodgy, but the most surprising thing of all is the outcome: the average change in eyebrow height 90 days post-treatment was 1.7mm. And this lift lasted for three months. How much is 1.7mm? Not a lot!

Considering Ultherapy treatments can set you back thousands of dollars or pounds, it is almost certainly not worth it.

MECHANICAL TREATMENTS

Thread-lifts

A 'thread-lift' is the use of special types of barbed-wire-type sutures (with cones replacing the hooks of the barbed wire), made of an absorbable material, that are inserted into the skin in areas of laxity to literally pull up and 'lift' the tissue. They are suggested to work in two ways: first, an early lifting action and second, a delayed regenerating action because the suture itself dissolves in the skin and works as a biostimulator (see page 265). Thread-lifts are meant to be a 'minimally invasive' way to achieve similar results to a surgical facelift. However, one systematic review found no substantial scientific evidence that thread-lift sutures have a long-lasting effect.[15] The lifting effect achieved is not only subtle, but also temporary, lasting between six and twelve months maximum, on average. The only two studies that showed a longer-lasting outcome were sponsored by the manufacturers of the actual threads.[16]

It would be truly amazing to achieve facelift results without surgery via a 30-minute in-office procedure and the marketing is powerful and captivating, so it is easy to see why patients are driven to get this treatment. The treatment itself costs a few thousand pounds and so the commercial incentives for the cosmetic doctors who perform it is high.

The bottom line: I don't recommend this treatment and advise my patients to avoid it.

Microneedling

Microneedling is known as 'percutaneous collagen induction' and is the use of small needles stuck into the dermis to stimulate the formation of new dermal collagen via scarless wound healing in a purely mechanical way (so without heat or light). Unlike ablative laser resurfacing and peels, the top of the skin (the epidermis) is not damaged, thus, theoretically, post-procedure 'downtime' should be minimal. For facial skin, the main suggested use is for the improvement of atrophic (pitted) acne scars and 'skin rejuvenation' (like fine lines/wrinkles) in general.

Microneedling requires a lot of repeated treatments to hopefully have a good effect and it takes months (or perhaps years) post-treatment to see an improvement, in keeping with the very slow turnover of collagen in the skin. Evidence suggests that the most significant improvements are not noticeable until 8–12 months post-treatment.[17] So be patient; this is not a treatment that you can judge just a few weeks after you have it. Much of the published research into microneedling has been undertaken by manufacturers of microneedling devices – so this suggests that these studies are inherently biased towards favouring positive outcomes. (Note that it is extremely difficult to do any clinical trials of microneedling because it is not possible to 'blind' the study because there is no placebo treatment it can be compared to.)

Though there is no scientific agreement on how deep the needle should go, it probably needs to go to a depth of at least 1.5mm into the skin in order to have any effect on dermal collagen – with 1.5mm and deeper, you would expect pinpoint bleeding (the epidermis is generally only 0.2mm thick) and that is the treatment 'end point'. You usually need 3–6 passes with a needle 1.5–3mm long to achieve this end point (ouch).[18]

There is no standard protocol for how often you need to have the treatment; in the literature, patients were treated between 1 and 12 times, with treatment intervals varying from 1 to 8 weeks.[19] There is some evidence to suggest superior results of doing weekly sessions for six weeks as a treatment course. Microneedling is painful when done correctly and will require the use of topical anaesthetic for most people. Downtime (redness and skin burning) lasts for about 48 hours post-treatment. It should not be done over active, inflamed acne or other inflamed skin rashes on the face, like rosacea or perioral dermatitis.

> **The bottom line**: If you want to do this, get it done by a doctor (because in most countries only doctors are allowed to microneedle beyond 2mm); don't DIY it at home (pointless waste of money), and don't do it if you have acne, perioral dermatitis or any other facial skin condition that is active.

The most important thing to remember when approaching any of these sorts of treatments is that they take time to make a difference, and often any change or improvement is subtle. You probably won't notice a dramatic improvement in skin sagging or laxity; the result you are aiming for is an increase in firmness or 'bounce' of the skin itself, your overall 'glow', not the structure of your face. As I have mentioned previously, if you have excess sagging skin or a lot of wrinkles and skin laxity, surgery is the only thing that will give you back a long-lasting defined jawline or truly 'tighten' the appearance of skin.

> **The bottom line**: The best uses of your time and money when it comes to skin rejuvenation include:

1. Wearing sunscreen daily when outdoors and actively avoiding sun exposure by wearing a hat and staying out of direct sunlight when outdoors.
2. Using tretinoin every night, consistently.
3. If you are female and in the region of menopause, considering HRT – discuss this with your doctor.
4. Considering investing in HA injections into your dermis perhaps every few years.
5. If you want to have an in-office treatment, investing your time and money in the most intense one that is suitable for you. Don't be scared of a little downtime if you want the most long-term benefits (though lifting sagging skin isn't one of them).
6. Above all, be patient and don't expect miracles.

Final Words

A few years ago, I had to buy a new car. My trusty Nissan Micra that saw me through my junior doctor years was on its last legs – it was time for an upgrade. I decided I wanted a similar compact car, so I googled 'best compact car' and was, as you can imagine, overwhelmed with options for different car brands, styles and, of course, price points. I narrowed it down to five brands by reading reviews and off I went to visit each dealership. I drove more cars – and listened to more sales pitches – than I ever want to again. I ended up buying the cheapest car on my list. And I loved it. Sure, I test drove a car that literally cost three times more (also a compact car) and yes it had lovely leather seats and lots of buttons on the dashboard that reminded me of the Starship *Enterprise*. But in the end, I realised that all compact cars are basically the same. The salesperson at the expensive dealership even admitted that the engine in the fancy expensive car is exactly the same as in the car I ended up buying.

Cars and cosmetic skincare products have a lot in common!

I hope you have found this book to be a wealth of information that will help you reach your skincare goals efficiently and effectively, saving you money and time searching for answers online.

Let's summarise the key points:

- If you have a skin problem – whether it is acne, rosacea, melasma or you just feel like your skin is 'dull' – get the correct diagnosis and a targeted management plan. The products recommended shouldn't cost more than the consultation with the doctor.

- Embrace basic, simple skincare: all you need is a cleanser (preferably oil-based and used once daily), a moisturiser for at night (preferably an ointment) and a sunscreen for the day (whichever you like).

- Don't buy expensive skincare products (unless you want to, of course) because, when it comes down to it, all the products are the same. The high price comes only from the packaging and the marketing – not the product itself.

- Stay away from products with fancy-sounding ingredients (anything derived from placenta or stem cells or made of gold or diamonds, for example) or extravagant marketing claims – all these things just increase the price of the product, not how well it works.

- Do not take advice about prescription treatments from someone who can't legally prescribe them; that encompasses most 'skinfluencers' on social media.

- The only truly evidence-based, science-backed topical treatment for combating the signs of ageing is retinoic acid. Everything else deemed an 'active' for fine lines, wrinkles, collagen regeneration or general 'anti-ageing' may do something, but there isn't enough high-quality evidence to support their use or the (often exorbitant) prices of the products themselves.

- The only evidence-based, science-backed topical treatment for hyperpigmentation and melasma is hydroquinone. It is safe and effective.

- 'Botox works every time' (as stated by Samantha in *Sex and the City*).

- Above all else, learn to love Vaseline.

In general, the overarching, practical, take-home message here is: **less is more**. Unless you have an actual skin problem that needs treatment, you can almost certainly use almost no skincare or very little. Many patients I see are trapped in a 'product use cycle': their skin is getting worse despite all the products they are using, so they add another product to try to make it better, get more irritation, then add in another product to fix that, leading to more irritation . . . and the cycle continues. The solution is to stop using all products for at least two weeks and then reintroduce the basics one at a time.

The bottom line: If you have a skin issue – acne, pigmentation, redness, overly dry or overly oily skin, or fine lines, whatever it may be – start with the correct diagnosis and ditch all unnecessary skincare.

SKINTELLIGENT TIP:

Don't get sucked in by FOMOOS

Do you have FOMOOS – Fear Of Missing Out On Skincare? A new product comes on the market and you just *have* to have it? I think this is a very serious problem.

One thing I say time and again is this: you are not going to develop skin issues or problems from *not* using a specific product, but you may develop one from using *too many* products. So keep it simple – less is more. Treat any problem you may have correctly and, hopefully, your days of FOMOOS will be behind you!

Your skin is very good at looking after itself. If you don't believe me, try it. Literally stop using all skincare for two weeks (unless you are on a specific doctor-prescribed treatment – consult your doctor before stopping that). And that means no skincare – including sunscreen (wear a hat or stay out of the sun if you are going to be outside and concerned about sun exposure). If you wear face make-up, try doing this during a time when you don't need to wear any, though this may not be practical for everyone. If you can't get around that, just use a basic (oil-based) cleanser to remove your make-up before bed and that's it. No moisturiser. The aim of this 'experiment' is to show you that skincare is generally unnecessary to keep your skin looking and feeling healthy.

The necessity of daily skincare for normal skin is an invention of Big Skincare, not medicine or science.

Appendix: How to Choose a Dermatologist

What's the difference between a consultant dermatologist and a 'specialist dermatologist'? What's a 'cosmetic dermatologist' or a 'laser doctor'? So and so is 'board certified by the American College of Cosmetic Dermatologists', but what does that actually mean?

I've said it before and I will say it again: dermatology is one of the only medical specialities where you will find people 'pretending' to be dermatologists and even calling themselves dermatologists when they are not. **'Dermatologist' is not a legally protected title.** The first thing to do when you find a dermatologist you are thinking of seeing is to go to the General Medical Council's website (www.gmc-uk.org) and check whether that doctor is on the 'specialist register for dermatology'. They should also have an individual GMC number (if you want to look me up, my GMC number is 7018298). If they are on the register, that means they are bona fide, fully trained consultant dermatologists who have completed a nationally recognised four-year training programme and passed the necessary exams (the equivalent of 'board-certified dermatologist' in the United States).

Even among consultant dermatologists, there is of course a huge amount of variability in knowledge and skill set. So how do you choose? In dermatology, as in most things, experience is the most important thing you are looking for. Forget the number of Instagram followers they have, their swanky clinic on Harley Street, what fancy university or hospital they trained at, how many celeb clients they claim to have had (remember a lot of these celeb clients are paid for their endorsement of said doctor), and even if they have written a book or two.

Experience comes from seeing patients so it can be difficult to figure out if your doctor has a lot or a little (age isn't actually a good indicator or even years in practice as many people work part time). I don't have a good answer for this, but looking at vetted legit doctor review sites like Doctify can be helpful.

Below are some of the red flags patients come and tell me about. If any of these attributes apply to the dermatologist you have seen, consider finding someone else:

- A dermatologist who does not take the time to listen to your concerns.
- A dermatologist who does not carefully examine your skin.
- A dermatologist who does not explain your treatment options and give you a fair estimate of cost for each option.
- A dermatologist who immediately tries to sell you an expensive form of treatment before discussing less expensive topical treatments first.
- A dermatologist who pushes you to buy an over-the-counter skincare product that is very expensive – doctors make commission on selling you these ridiculously expensive lotions and potions. Do not fall for it. A doctor cannot earn commission from selling prescription medications to you – that is illegal and unethical.
- A dermatologist who tells you that you 'have to have Botox' or you 'have to have filler' – no one needs Botox or filler, ever.
- A dermatologist who does not suggest a 'cooling off period' prior to a cosmetic treatment.
- A dermatologist who 'guarantees' results from a procedure or intervention.
- A dermatologist who tells you they can perform 'scarless' surgery.
- A dermatologist who prescribes you a treatment but does not tell you the actual diagnosis. A treatment should be targeted to a specific diagnosis, so if the doctor you see can't give you the diagnosis and explain it to you, do not use the treatment.

Acknowledgements

A massive thank you to the team at Vermilion, especially Sam Jackson, who recognised the need for this book and pushed to get others to see it too, and Julia Kellaway, for her amazing editorial skills!

To my parents, of course, to whom this book is dedicated. Your support over the past 41 years has allowed me to chase my goals and think big.

To all my patients – past, present and future – for inspiring me to do what I do (and keep on doing it) every day.

To my Instagram family – for following along on my journey and keeping me true to myself. Thank you, especially, to Team Trifle!

And thank you to all my incredible friends who have supported me (and put up with me) throughout this process: my Dubai family – Caroline, David, Mimi, Max, Kyle, Mousse, Maple and Pie – I am grateful and honoured to be part of the LaBoosh family. EJ (my MVP), Sophie, Nasrah, Barbara, and Ty.

And in London: Samer for the power walks and wisdom, Soga and the whole team at London Medical, Usamah, Samantha, Sobi, Jill and Mark and your family, Dr Ed (thanks for letting me have time off work to write this!). A big thank you to Menno for helping me stay on track. Thank you to Sammi who set me on the social media path and for Julia who is carrying on the torch, keeping it bright and vibrant!

And, finally, thank you to Dr Albert Kligman: your tremendous work has inspired me to be better and think outside the dermatology box. I would have moved to Pennsylvania to have had the chance to work with you.

References

Introduction

1 Statista Research Department. Global skin care market size 2012–2025. 2 Feb 2022. Available from https://www.statista.com/statistics/254612/global-skin-care-market-size.

Part 1: How Skin Works

1 Balin AK, Kligman AM (eds). *Aging and the Skin*. Raven Press, 1989.
2 Buglass L. This is how much the average woman spends on skincare. *Woman & Home*. 16 May 2019. Available from https://www.womanandhome.com/beauty/beauty-news/average-woman-spends-skincare-321315.

Chapter 1: The Structure of the Skin

1 Akdeniz M, Gabriel S, Lichterfeld-Kottner A et al. Transepidermal water loss in healthy adults: a systematic review and meta-analysis update. *Br J Dermatol.* 2018 Nov;179(5):1049–1055; Kottner J, Lichterfeld A, Blume-Peytavi U. Transepidermal water loss in young and aged healthy humans: a systematic review and meta-analysis. *Arch Dermatol Res.* 2013 May;305(4):315–323.
2 Elias PM, Feingold KR (eds). *Skin Barrier*. CRC Press, 2006: first edition.
3 Kligman AM. Corneobiology and corneotherapy – a final chapter. *Int J Cosmet Sci.* 2011 Jun;33(3):197–209.
4 Rawlings AV, Scott IR, Harding CR et al. Stratum corneum moisturization at the molecular level. *J Invest Dermatol.* 1994 Nov;103(5):731–741.
5 Verdier-Sévrain S, Bonté F. Skin hydration: a review on its molecular mechanisms. *J Cosmet Dermatol.* 2007 Jun;6(2):75–82.
6 Ibid.
7 Elias PM. Structure and function of the stratum corneum extracellular matrix. *J Invest Dermatol.* 2012 Sep;132(9):2131–2133.

8 Surber C, Humbert P, Abels C et al. The acid mantle: a myth or an essential part of skin health? *Curr Probl Dermatol.* 2018;54:1–10.

9 Elias PM, Sun R, Eder AR et al. Treating atopic dermatitis at the source: corrective barrier repair therapy based upon new pathogenic insights. *Expert Rev Dermatol.* 2013 Feb;8(1):27–36.

10 van Smeden J, Bouwstra JA. Stratum corneum lipids: their role for the skin barrier function in healthy subjects and atopic dermatitis patients. *Curr Probl Dermatol.* 2016;49:8–26.

11 Rawlings AV, Matts PJ. Stratum corneum moisturization at the molecular level: an update in relation to the dry skin cycle. *J Invest Dermatol.* 2005 Jun;124(6):1099–1110; Rawlings AV, Scott IR, Harding CR et al. Stratum corneum moisturization at the molecular level. *J Invest Dermatol.* 1994 Nov;103(5):731–741.

12 Fuchs E. Skin stem cells: rising to the surface. *J Cell Biol.* 2008 Jan;180(2):273–284.

13 Scheuplein RJ, Bronaugh RL. Percutaneous absorption. In: Goldsmith LA (ed). *Biochemistry and Physiology of the Skin.* Oxford University Press, 1983: 1255–1295.

14 Sahle FF, Gebre-Mariam T, Dobner B et al. Skin diseases associated with the depletion of stratum corneum lipids and stratum corneum lipid substitution therapy. *Skin Pharmacol Physiol.* 2015;28(1):42–55.

15 Gonzales KAU, Fuchs E. Skin and its regenerative powers: an alliance between stem cells and their niche. *Dev Cell.* 2017 Nov;43(4): 387–401.

16 James WDI, Elston DM, Treat J et al. *Andrews' Diseases of the Skin: Clinical Dermatology.* Elsevier, 2020: thirteenth edition.

17 Kottner J, Lichterfeld A, Blume-Peytavi U. Transepidermal water loss in young and aged healthy humans: a systematic review and meta-analysis. *Arch Dermatol Res.* 2013 May;305(4):315–323.

18 Fisher GJ, Varani J, Voorhees JJ. Looking older: fibroblast collapse and therapeutic implications. *Arch Dermatol.* 2008;144(5):666–672.

Chapter 2: The Myth of the Skin 'Type'

1 Roberts WE. Skin type classification systems old and new. *Dermatol Clin.* 2009 Oct;27(4):529–533, viii.

2 Sakuma TH, Maibach HI. Oily skin: an overview. *Skin Pharmacol Physiol.* 2012;25(5):227–235.

3 Ibid.

4 Paula's Choice Skincare. Alcohol in skincare: the facts. Available from https://www.paulaschoice-eu.com/alcohol-in-skincare-the-facts.

5 Kligman AM, Shelley WB. An investigation of the biology of the human sebaceous gland. *J Invest Dermatol.* 1958;30:99–125.

6 Smith K, Thiboutot D. Thematic review series: skin lipids. Sebaceous gland lipids: friend or foe? *J Lipid Res.* 2008;49:271–281.

7 Altemus M, Rao B, Dhabhar FS et al. Stress-induced changes in skin barrier function in healthy women. *J Invest Dermatol.* 2001 Aug;117(2):309–317.

8 Akdeniz M, Tomova-Simitchieva T, Dobos G et al. Does dietary fluid intake affect skin hydration in healthy humans? A systematic literature review. *Skin Res Technol.* 2018; 24: 459–465.

9 Madison KC. Barrier function of the skin: 'la raison d'être' of the epidermis. *J Invest Dermatol.* 2003 Aug;121(2):231–341.

10 Esacalas-Taberner J, Gonzalez-Guerra E, Guerra-Tapia A. Sensitive skin: a complex syndrome. *Actas Dermosifiliogr.* 2011;102(8): 563–571.

11 Misery L. Sensitive skin and rosacea: a nosologic framework. *Annales de dermatolgie et de venereology.* 2011;138:S207–S210; Misery L. Neuropsychiatric factors in sensitive skin. *Clinics in Dermatology.* 2017;35:281–284.

Chapter 3: How Skin Changes as We Age

1 Akdeniz M, Tomova-Simitchieva T, Dobos G et al. Does dietary fluid intake affect skin hydration in healthy humans? A systematic literature review. *Skin Res Technol.* 2018;24:459–465; Kottner J, Lichterfeld A, Blume-Peytavi U. Transepidermal water loss in young and aged healthy humans: a systematic review and meta-analysis. *Arch Dermatol Res.* 2013 May;305(4):315–323.

2 Wang Z, Man MQ, Li T et al. Aging-associated alterations in epidermal function and their clinical significance. *Aging (Albany NY).* 2020 Mar;12(6):5551–5565.

3 Elias PM, Ghadially R. The aged epidermal permeability barrier: basis for functional abnormalities. *Clin Geriatr Med.* 2002 Feb;18(1):103–120, vii; Ghadially R, Brown BE, Sequeira-Martin SM et al. The aged epidermal permeability barrier. Structural, functional, and lipid biochemical abnormalities in humans and a senescent murine model. *J Clin Invest.* 1995 May;95(5): 2281–2290.

4 Saint-Léger D, François AM, Lévêque JL et al. Stratum corneum lipids in skin xerosis. *Dermatologica.* 1989;178(3):151–155.

5 Fisher GJ, Varani J, Voorhees JJ. Looking older: fibroblast collapse and therapeutic implications. *Arch Dermatol.* 2008;144(5): 666–672.

6 Handler MZ, Goldberg DJ. Neocollagenesis. In: Goldberg DJ (ed). *Dermal Fillers*. Karger Publishers, 2018;vol. 4:27–35.

7 Ibid.

8 Balin AK, Kligman AM (eds). *Aging and the Skin*. Raven Press, 1989.

9 Shuster S, Black MM, McVitie E. The influence of age and sex on skin thickness, skin collagen and density. *Br J Dermatol*. 1975 Dec;93(6):639–643.

10 Marcos-Garcés V, Molina Aguilar P, Bea Serrano C et al. Age-related dermal collagen changes during development, maturation and ageing – a morphometric and comparative study. *J Anat*. 2014 Jul;225(1):98–108.

11 Haydont V, Bernard BA, Fortunel NO. Age-related evolutions of the dermis: clinical signs, fibroblast and extracellular matrix dynamics. *Mech Ageing Dev*. 2019 Jan;177:150–156.

12 Lambros V. Observations on periorbital and midface aging. *Plast Reconstr Surg*. 2007 Oct;120(5):1367–1376.

13 Haydont V, Bernard BA, Fortunel NO. Age-related evolutions of the dermis: clinical signs, fibroblast and extracellular matrix dynamics. *Mech Ageing Dev*. 2019 Jan;177:150–156.

Part 2: How Skincare Works (Or Doesn't)

1 Bercovitch L, Perlis CS (eds). *Dermatoethics*. Springer, 2021.

2 Tungate M. *Branded Beauty: How marketing changed the way we look*. Kogan Page, 2011.

3 Ibid.

4 Bigby M. Snake oil for the 21st century. *Arch Dermatol*. 1998 Dec;134(12):1512–1514.

Chapter 4: Facial Cleansers and Moisturisers

1 Maarouf M, Saberian C, Shi VY. Myths, truths, and clinical relevance of comedogenicity product labeling. *JAMA Dermatol*. 2018 Oct;154(10):1131–1132.

2 Katoulis AC, Kakepis EM, Kintziou H et al. Comedogenicity of cosmetics: a review. *JEADV*. 1996 Sept;7(2):115–119.

3 Kligman AM, Mills OH Jr. 'Acne cosmetica'. *Arch Dermatol*. 1972 Dec;106(6):843–850.

4 Mills OH Jr, Kligman AM. A human model for assessing comedogenic substances. *Arch Dermatol*. 1982 Nov;118(11):903–905.

5 Ibid.

6   Draelos ZD. The effect of a daily facial cleanser for normal to oily skin on the skin barrier of subjects with acne. *Cutis.* 2006 Jul;78(1 Suppl):34–40.

7   Kligman AM. Petrolatum is not comedogenic in rabbits or humans: a critical reappraisal of the rabbit ear assay and the concept of 'acne cosmetica'. *J Soc Cosmet Chem.* 1996;47:41–48.

8   Hosokawa K, Taima H, Kikuchi M et al. Rubbing the skin when removing makeup cosmetics is a major factor that worsens skin conditions in atopic dermatitis patients. *J Cosmet Dermatol.* 2021 Jun;20(6):1915–1922; Li G, Wang B, Zhao Z et al. Excessive cleansing: an underestimating risk factor of rosacea in Chinese population. *Arch Dermatol Res.* 2021 May;313(4):225–234.

9   Solomon BA, Shalita AR. Effects of detergents on acne. *Clin Dermatol.* 1996 Jan–Feb;14(1):95–99.

10 Ananthapadmanabhan KP, Moore DJ, Subramanyan K et al. Cleansing without compromise: the impact of cleansers on the skin barrier and the technology of mild cleansing. *Dermatol Ther.* 2004;17(Suppl 1):16–25.

11 Hosokawa K, Taima H, Kikuchi M et al. Rubbing the skin when removing makeup cosmetics is a major factor that worsens skin conditions in atopic dermatitis patients. *J Cosmet Dermatol.* 2021 Jun;20(6):1915–1922.

12 Businesswire. P&G announces fourth quarter and fiscal year 2020 results. 30 Jul 2020. Available from https://www.business wire.com/news/home/20200730005458/en/PG-Announces-Fourth-Quarter-and-Fiscal-Year-2020-Results.

13 Kligman AM. Corneobiology and corneotherapy – a final chapter. *Int J Cosmet Sci.* 2011 Jun;33(3):197–209.

14 Comaish JS, Greener JS. The inhibiting effect of soft paraffin on the Köbner response in psoriasis. *Br J Dermatol.* 1976 Feb;94(2):195–200.

15 Kligman LH, Kligman AM. Petrolatum and other hydrophobic emollients reduce UVB-induced damage. *J Dermatolog Treat.* 1992 Jan;3(1):3–7.

16 Held E, Lund H, Agner T. Effect of different moisturizers on SLS-irritated human skin. *Con Derm.* 2001 Apr;44(4):229–234.

17 Kligman AM. Petrolatum is not comedogenic in rabbits or humans: a critical reappraisal of the rabbit ear assay and the concept of 'acne cosmetica'. *J Soc Cosmet Chem.* 1996;47:41–48.

18 Held E, Sveinsdóttir S, Agner T. Effect of long-term use of moisturizer on skin hydration, barrier function and susceptibility to irritants. *Acta Derm Venereol.* 1999 Jan;79(1):49–51.

19 Serup J. A double-blind comparison of two creams containing urea as the active ingredient. Assessment of efficacy and

side-effects by non-invasive techniques and a clinical scoring scheme. *Acta Derm Venereol Suppl (Stockh)*. 1992;177:34–43.

20 Serup J, Winther A, Blichmann CW. Effects of repeated application of a moisturizer. *Acta Derm Venereol*. 1989;69(5):457–459.

21 Draelos ZD. An evaluation of prescription device moisturisers. *J Cosmet Dermatol*. 2009;8:40–43; Miller DW, Koch SB, Yentzer BA et al. An over-the-counter moisturizer is as clinically effective as, and more cost-effective than, prescription barrier creams in the treatment of children with mild to moderate AD: a randomized, controlled trial. *J Drugs Dermatol*. 2011;10:531–537.

22 Loden M, Buraczewska I, Halvarsson K. Facial anti-wrinkle cream: Influence of product presentation on effectiveness: A randomised and controlled study. *Ski Res Technol*. 2007;13(2):189–194.

23 Agero AL, Verallo-Rowell VM. A randomized double-blind controlled trial comparing extra virgin coconut oil with mineral oil as a moisturizer for mild to moderate xerosis. *Dermatitis*. 2004 Sep;15(3):109–116; Evangelista MT, Abad-Casintahan F, Lopez-Villafuerte L. The effect of topical virgin coconut oil on SCORAD index, transepidermal water loss, and skin capacitance in mild to moderate pediatric atopic dermatitis: a randomized, double-blind, clinical trial. *Int J Dermatol*. 2014 Jan;53(1):100–108; Nangia S, Paul VK, Deorari AK et al. Topical oil application and transepidermal water loss in preterm very low birth weight infants – a randomized trial. *J Trop Pediatr*. 2015 Dec;61(6):414–420.

Chapter 5: Sunscreen

1 Samuel M, Brooke RC, Hollis S et al. Interventions for photodamaged skin. *Cochrane Database Syst Rev*. 2005 Jan;(1):CD001782.

2 Petersen B, Wulf HC. Application of sunscreen – theory and reality. *Photodermatol Photoimmunol Photomed*. 2014 Apr–Jun;30(2–3):96–101.

3 Ludriksone L, Elsner P. Adverse reactions to sunscreens. *Curr Probl Dermatol*. 2021;55:223–235.

4 Chen W, He M, Xie L et al. The optimal cleansing method for the removal of sunscreen: water, cleanser or cleansing oil? *J Cosmet Dermatol*. 2020 Jan;19(1):180–184.

5 British Association of Dermatologists. Sunscreen fact sheet. 2013. Available from https://www.bad.org.uk/page.aspx?sitesectionid=1020.

6 Ibid.

7 Rungan**anchai C, Silpa-Archa N, Wongpraparut C et al. Sunscreen application to the face persists beyond 2 hours in indoor

workers: an open-label trial. *J Dermatolog Treat*. 2019 Aug;30(5): 483–486.

8   COSlaw.eu. Sunscreen products and claims: a guidance to the EU regulatory framework. 30 Jun 2021. Available from https:// www.coslaw.eu/sunscreen-products-and-claims-a-guidance-to-the-eu-regulatory-framework.

9   Matta MK, Zusterzeel R, Pilli NR et al. Effect of sunscreen application under maximal use conditions on plasma concentration of sunscreen active ingredients: a randomized clinical trial. *JAMA*. 2019 Jun;321(21):2082–2091; Matta MK, Florian J, Zusterzeel R et al. Effect of sunscreen application on plasma concentration of sunscreen active ingredients: a randomized clinical trial. *JAMA*. 2020 Jan;323(3):256–267.

10 Williams JD, Maitra P, Atillasoy E et al. SPF 100+ sunscreen is more protective against sunburn than SPF 50+ in actual use: results of a randomized, double-blind, split-face, natural sunlight exposure clinical trial. *J Am Acad Dermatol*. 2018 May;78(5):902–910.e2.

11 Duteil L, Queille-Roussel C, Lacour JP et al. Short-term exposure to blue light emitted by electronic devices does not worsen melasma. *J Am Acad Dermatol*. 2020 Sep;83(3):913–914.

12 Kleinpenning MM, Smits T, Frunt MH et al. Clinical and histological effects of blue light on normal skin. *Photodermatol Photoimmunol Photomed*. 2010;26(1):16–21.

13 Dumbuya H, Grimes PE, Lynch S et al. Impact of iron-oxide containing formulations against visible light-induced skin pigmentation in skin of color individuals. *J Drugs Dermatol*. 2020 Jul;19(7):712–717.

Chapter 6: Skincare Products You Don't Need

1   Draelos ZD. Cosmeceuticals: what's real, what's not. *Dermatol Clin*. 2019 Jan;37(1):107–115.

2   Ng JNC, Wanitphakdeedecha R, Yan C. Efficacy of home-use light-emitting diode device at 637 and 854-nm for facial rejuvenation: a split-face pilot study. *J Cosmet Dermatol*. 2020 Sep;19(9): 2288–2294.

3   MarketsandMarkets. Examine collagen market is projected to reach $4.6 billion by 2023. WhaTech. 9 May 2021. Available from https://www.whatech.com/markets-research/medical/697445-collagen-market-is-projected-to-reach-4-6-billion-by-2023.

4   Alam M, Walter AJ, Geisler A et al. Association of facial exercise with the appearance of aging. *JAMA Dermatol*. 2018 Mar;154(3): 365–367.

5   Kligman AM. Cosmetics. A dermatologist looks to the future: promises and problems. *Dermatol Clin.* 2000 Oct;18(4): 699–709.

Part 3: Unravelling Big Skincare Ingredient Claims

1   Varagur K. The skincare con. The Outline. 30 Jan 2018. Available from https://theoutline.com/post/3151/the-skincare-con-glossier-drunk-elephant-biologique-recherche-p50.

2   Kligman AM. Cosmetics. A dermatologist looks to the future: promises and problems. *Dermatol Clin.* 2000 Oct;18(4):699–709.

3   Kligman D. Cosmeceuticals. *Dermatol Clin.* 2000 Oct;18(4): 609–615.

4   Elias PM, Feingold KR (eds). *Skin Barrier.* CRC Press, 2006: first edition.

5   Pouillot A, Dayan N, Polla AS et al. The stratum corneum: a double paradox. *J Cosmet Dermatol.* 2008 Jun;7(2):143–148.

6   Bos JD, Meinardi MM. The 500 Dalton rule for the skin penetration of chemical compounds and drugs. *Exp Dermatol.* 2000 Jun;9(3): 165–169.

7   Ibid.

8   Motosko CC, Ault AK, Kimberly LL et al. Analysis of spin in the reporting of studies of topical treatments of photoaged skin. *J Am Acad Dermatol.* 2019 Feb;80(2):516–522.e12.

9   Ibid.

Chapter 7: Vitamin A

1   Kligman LH. Photoaging. Manifestations, prevention, and treatment. *Dermatol Clin.* 1986 Jul;4(3):517–528; Kligman AM, Fulton JE Jr, Plewig G. Topical vitamin A acid in acne vulgaris. *Arch Dermatol.* 1969 Apr;99(4):469–476.

2   Griffiths CE, Russman AN, Majmudar G et al. Restoration of collagen formation in photodamaged human skin by tretinoin (retinoic acid). *N Engl J Med.* 1993 Aug;329(8):530–535.

3   Kligman LH. Photoaging. Manifestations, prevention, and treatment. *Dermatol Clin.* 1986 Jul;4(3):517–528.

4   Mukherjee S, Date A, Patravale V et al. Retinoids in the treatment of skin aging: an overview of clinical efficacy and safety. *Clin Interv Aging.* 2006;1(4):327–348.

5   Renova FDA drug data. Reference ID: 3524057. Approved by FDA 31 Aug 2000.

6   Renova (tretinoin cream) leaflet. Available from https://www.accessdata.fda.gov/drugsatfda_docs/label/2014/021108s015lbl.pdf.

7   Renova FDA drug data. Reference ID: 3524057. Approved by FDA 31 Aug 2000.

8   Spierings NMK. Evidence for the efficacy of over-the-counter vitamin A cosmetic productions in the improvement of facial skin aging: a systematic review. *J Clin Aesthet Dermatol.* 2021;14(9): 33–40.

9   Kligman AM. Guidelines for the use of topical tretinoin (Retin-A) for photoaged skin. *J Am Acad Dermatol.* 1989 Sep;21(3 Pt 2): 650–654.

10   Griffiths CEM, Kang S, Ellis CN et al. Two concentrations of topical tretinoin (retinoic acid) cause similar improvement of photoaging but different degree of irritation. *Arch Dermatol* 1995;131:1037–1044; Renova (tretinoin cream) leaflet. Available from https://www.accessdata.fda.gov/drugsatfda_docs/label/2014/021108s015lbl.pdf.

11   Didierjean L, Carraux P, Grand D et al. Topical retinaldehyde increases skin content of retinoic acid and exerts biologic activity in mouse skin. *J Invest Dermatol* 1996;107:714–719.

12   Kligman AM. Guidelines for the use of topical tretinoin (Retin-A) for photoaged skin. *J Am Acad Dermatol.* 1989 Sep;21(3 Pt 2): 650–654.

13   Ibid.

14   Bhawan J, Gonzalez-Serva A, Nehal K et al. Effects of tretinoin on photodamaged skin. A histologic study. *Arch Dermatol.* 1991 May;127(5):666–6672; Bhawan J. Short- and long-term histologic effects of topical tretinoin on photodamaged skin. *Int J Dermatol.* 1998 Apr;37(4):286–292; Kligman AM. Guidelines for the use of topical tretinoin (Retin-A) for photoaged skin. *J Am Acad Dermatol.* 1989 Sep;21(3 Pt 2):650–654.

Chapter 8: Hydroquinone

1   Tse TW. Hydroquinone for skin lightening: safety profile, duration of use and when should we stop? *J Dermatolog Treat.* 2010 Sep;21(5):272–275; Draelos ZD. Skin lightening preparations and the hydroquinone controversy. *Dermatol Ther.* 2007;20: 308–313.

2   Rendon M. Melasma and postinflammatory hyperpigmentation. *Cosmet Dermatol*. 2003;16:9–15.

3   Tse TW. Hydroquinone for skin lightening: safety profile, duration of use and when should we stop? *J Dermatolog Treat*. 2010 Sep;21(5):272–275.

4   Petit A. Skin lightening and its motives: a historical overview. *Ann Dermatol Venereol*. 2019 May;146(5):399–409.

5   Ibid.

6   Levitt J. The safety of hydroquinone: a dermatologist's response to the 2006 Federal Register. *J Am Acad Dermatol*. 2007 Nov;57(5): 854–872.

7   Tse TW. Hydroquinone for skin lightening: safety profile, duration of use and when should we stop? *J Dermatolog Treat*. 2010 Sep;21(5):272–275.

8   Levitt J. The safety of hydroquinone: a dermatologist's response to the 2006 Federal Register. *J Am Acad Dermatol*. 2007 Nov;57(5): 854–872.

9   Ibid.

10 Torok H, Taylor S, Baumann L et al. A large 12-month extension study of an 8-week trial to evaluate the safety and efficacy of triple combination (TC) cream in melasma patients previously treated with TC cream or one of its dyads. *J Drugs Dermatol*. 2005;4:592–597; FDA Triluma approval summary document. 2002. Available from https://www.accessdata.fda.gov/drugsatfda_docs/nda/2002/21-112_TRI-Luma_medr_P2.pdf.

11 DeCaprio AP. The toxicology of hydroquinone – relevance to occupational and environmental exposure. *Crit Rev Toxicol*. 1999 May;29(3):283–330.

12 Lueangarun S, Namboonlue C, Tempark T. Postinflammatory and rebound hyperpigmentation as a complication after treatment efficacy of telangiectatic melasma with 585 nanometers Q-switched Nd: YAG laser and 4% hydroquinone cream in skin phototypes III–V. *J Cosmet Dermatol*. 2021 Jun;20(6):1700–1708.

13 Torok H, Taylor S, Baumann L et al. A large 12-month extension study of an 8-week trial to evaluate the safety and efficacy of triple combination (TC) cream in melasma patients previously treated with TC cream or one of its dyads. *J Drugs Dermatol*. 2005;4:592–597.

14 Kligman AM, Willis I. A new formula for depigmenting human skin. *Arch Dermatol*. 1975;111:40–48.

15 Spierings, NMK. Melasma: A critical analysis of clinical trials investigating treatment modalities published in the past 10 years. *J Cosmetic Dermatol*. 2020 Jun;19(6):1284–1289.

16 Ibid.

Chapter 9: Vitamin C

1 Bartholomew M. James Lind's treatise of the scurvy (1753). *Postgrad Med J*. 2002 Nov;78(925):695–696.

2 McMullen RL. *Antioxidants and the Skin*. CRC Press, 2019: second edition.

3 Pham-Huy LA, He H, Pham-Huy C. Free radicals, antioxidants in disease and health. *Int J Biomed Sci*. 2008;4(2):89–96.

4 Ibid.

5 Ibid.

6 Pinnell SR. Cutaneous photodamage, oxidative stress, and topical antioxidant protection. *J Am Acad Dermatol*. 2003 Jan;48(1):1–19; quiz:20–2.

7 Draelos ZD. Cosmeceuticals: what's real, what's not. *Dermatol Clin*. 2019 Jan;37(1):107–115.

8 Nusgens BV, Humbert P, Rougier A et al. Topically applied vitamin C enhances the mRNA level of collagens I and III, their processing enzymes and tissue inhibitor of matrix metalloproteinase 1 in the human dermis. *J Invest Dermatol*. 2001 Jun;116(6):853–859.

Chapter 10: Acids

1 Rajanala S, Vashi NA. Cleopatra and sour milk – the ancient practice of chemical peeling. *JAMA Dermatol*. 2017;153(10):1006.

2 Thibault PK, Wlodarczyk J, Wenck A. A double-blind randomized clinical trial on the effectiveness of a daily glycolic acid 5% formulation in the treatment of photoaging. *Dermatol Surg*. 1998 May;24(5):573–577; discussion:577–578.

3 Pierard GE, Kligman AM, Stoudemayer T et al. Comparative effects of retinoic acid, glycolic acid and a lipophilic derivative of salicylic acid on photodamaged epidermis. *Dermatology*. 1999;199(1):50–53.

4 Tang SC, Yang JH. Dual effects of alpha-hydroxy acids on the skin. *Molecules*. 2018 Apr;23(4):863.

5 Fartasch M, Teal J, Menon GK. Mode of action of glycolic acid on human stratum corneum: ultrastructural and functional evaluation of the epidermal barrier. *Arch Dermatol Res*. 1997 Jun;289(7):404–409.

6 Leyden JJ, McGinley KJ, Mills OH et al. Effects of sulfur and salicylic acid in a shampoo base in the treatment of dandruff: a double-blind study using corneocyte counts and clinical grading. *Cutis*. 1987 Jun;39(6):557–561.

7 Ibid.

8   Searle T, Ali FR, Al-Niaimi F. The versatility of azelaic acid in dermatology. *J Dermatolog Treat*. 2020 Aug;4:1–11; Plewig G, Melnik B, Chen W. *Plewig and Kligman's Acne and Rosaea*. Springer, 2019: fourth edition.

9   Zhu J, Tang X, Jia Y et al. Applications and delivery mechanisms of hyaluronic acid used for topical/transdermal delivery – a review. *Int J Pharm*. 2020 Mar;578:119127.

10 Wu X, Zhang H, He S et al. Improving dermal delivery of hyaluronic acid by ionic liquids for attenuating skin dehydration. *Int J Biol Macromol*. 2020 May;150:528–535.

11 Lubart R, Yariv I, Fixler D et al. Topical hyaluronic acid facial cream with new micronized molecule technology effectively penetrates and improves facial skin quality: results from *In-vitro*, *Ex-vivo*, and *In-vivo* (open-label) studies. *J Clin Aesthet Dermatol*. 2019 Oct;12(10):39–44.

Chapter 11: Other Common Cosmetic Ingredients

1   Kligman AM. Cosmetics. A dermatologist looks to the future: promises and problems. *Dermatol Clin*. 2000 Oct;18(4):699–709.

2   Spierings NMK. Cosmetic commentary: Is bakuchiol the new 'skincare hero'? *J Cosmet Dermatol*. 2020 Dec;19(12):3208–3209.

3   Spierings NMK. Evidence for the efficacy of over-the-counter vitamin A cosmetic productions in the improvement of facial skin aging: a systematic review. *J Clin Aesthet Dermatol*. 2021;14(9):33–40.

4   Chaudhuri RK, Bojanowski K. Bakuchiol: A retinol-like functional compound revealed by gene expression profiling and clinically proven to have anti-aging effects. *Int J Cosmet Sci*. 2014;36(3):221–230.

5   Dhaliwal S, Rybak I, Ellis SR et al. Prospective, randomized, double-blind assessment of topical bakuchiol and retinol for facial photoageing. *Br J Dermatol*. 2019;180(2):289–296.

6   Spierings NMK. Cosmetic commentary: Is bakuchiol the new 'skincare hero'? *J Cosmet Dermatol*. 2020 Dec;19(12):3208–3209.

7   Draelos ZD, Matsubara A, Smiles K. The effect of 2% niacinamide on facial sebum production. *J Cosmet Laser Ther*. 2006 Jun;8(2):96–101; Fu JJ, Hillebrand GG, Raleigh P et al. A randomized, controlled comparative study of the wrinkle reduction benefits of a cosmetic niacinamide/peptide/retinyl propionate product regimen vs. a prescription 0.02% tretinoin product regimen. *Br J Dermatol*. 2010 Mar;162(3):647–54; Navarrete-Solís J, Castanedo-Cázares JP, Torres-Álvarez B et al. A double-blind, randomized clinical trial of niacinamide 4% versus hydroquinone 4% in the

treatment of melasma. *Dermatol Res Pract*. 2011;2011:379173; Walocko FM, Eber AE, Keri JE et al. The role of nicotinamide in acne treatment. *Dermatol Ther*. 2017 Sep;30(5); Namazi MR. Nicotinamide in dermatology: a capsule summary. *Int J Dermatol*. 2007 Dec;46(12):1229–1231; Soma Y, Kashima M, Imaizumi A et al. Moisturizing effects of topical nicotinamide on atopic dry skin. *Int J Dermatol*. 2005 Mar;44(3):197–202.

8   Walocko FM, Eber AE, Keri JE et al. The role of nicotinamide in acne treatment. *Dermatol Ther*. 2017 Sep;30(5).

9   Soma Y, Kashima M, Imaizumi A et al. Moisturizing effects of topical nicotinamide on atopic dry skin. *Int J Dermatol*. 2005 Mar;44(3):197–202.

10   Bercovitch L, Perlis CS (eds). *Dermatoethics*. Springer, 2021.

Part 4: How to Treat the Most Common Facial Skin Diseases

1   All Party Parliamentary Group on Skin. The psychological and social impact of skin diseases on people's lives. 2013. Available from https://www.appgs.co.uk/publication/view/the-psychological-and-social-impact-of-skin-diseases-on-peoples-lives-final-report-2013/.

2   Lukaviciute L, Ganceviciene R, Navickas P et al. Anxiety, depression, and suicidal ideation amongst patients with facial dermatoses (acne, rosacea, perioral dermatitis, and folliculitis) in Lithuania. *Dermatology*. 2020;236(4):314–322.

Chapter 12: Acne Vulgaris

1   Kligman AM. An overview of acne. *J Invest Dermatol*. 1974 Mar;62(3):268–287.

2   Scholz CFP, Kilian M. The natural history of cutaneous propionibacteria, and reclassification of selected species within the genus Propionibacterium to the proposed novel genera Acidipropionibacterium gen. nov., Cutibacterium gen. nov. and Pseudopropionibacterium gen. nov. *Int J Syst Evol Microbiol*. 2016 Nov;66(11):4422–4432; Dréno B, Pécastaings S, Corvec S et al. Cutibacterium acnes (Propionibacterium acnes) and acne vulgaris: a brief look at the latest updates. *J Eur Acad Dermatol Venereol*. 2018 Jun;32(Suppl 2):5–14.

3   Tan AU, Schlosser BJ, Paller AS. A review of diagnosis and treatment of acne in adult female patients. *Int J Womens Dermatol*. 2017;4(2):56–71.

4 Orentreich N, Durr NP. The natural evolution of comedones into inflammatory papules and pustules. *J Inv Dermatol.* 1974;62(3): 316–320.

5 Bershad S, Poulin YP, Berson DS et al. Topical retinoids in the treatment of acne vulgaris. *Cutis.* 1999 Aug;64(2 Suppl):8–20; quiz:21–3.

6 Grosshans E, Marks R, Mascaro JM et al. Evaluation of clinical efficacy and safety of adapalene 0.1% gel versus tretinoin 0.025% gel in the treatment of acne vulgaris, with particular reference to the onset of action and impact on quality of life. *Br J Dermatol.* 1998 Oct;139(Suppl 52):26–33.

7 Tolaymat L, Dearborn H, Zito PM. Adapalene. *StatPearls* [Internet]. 2022 Jan.

8 Kolli SS, Pecone D, Pona A et al. Topical retinoids in acne vulgaris: a systematic review. *Am J Clin Dermatol.* 2019 Jun;20(3): 345–365.

9 Barbaric J, Abbott R, Posadzki P et al. Light therapies for acne. *Cochrane Database Syst Rev.* 2016 Sep;9(9):CD007917.

10 Bek-Thomsen M, Lomholt HB, Kilian M. Acne is not associated with yet-uncultured bacteria. *J Clin Microbiol.* 2008 Oct;46(10): 3355–3360.

11 Arowojolu AO, Gallo MF, Lopez LM et al. Combined oral contraceptive pills for treatment of acne. *Cochrane Database Syst Rev.* 2012 Jul;(7):CD004425.

12 Ruan X, Kubba A, Aguilar A et al. Use of cyproterone acetate/ ethinylestradiol in polycystic ovary syndrome: rationale and practical aspects. *Eur J Contracept Reprod Health Care.* 2017 Jun;22(3):183–190.

13 Layton AM, Eady EA, Whitehouse H et al. Oral spironolactone for acne vulgaris in adult females: a hybrid systematic review. *Am J Clin Dermatol.* 2017 Apr;18(2):169–191; Trivedi MK, Shinkai K, Murase JE. A review of hormone-based therapies to treat adult acne vulgaris in women. *Int J Womens Dermatol.* 2017 Mar;3(1): 44–52.

14 Yamamoto A, Takenouchi K, Ito M. Impaired water barrier function in acne vulgaris. *Arch Dermatol Res.* 1995;287(2):214–218.

15 Swinyer LJ, Swinyer TA, Britt MR. Topical agents alone in acne. A blind assessment study. *JAMA.* 1980 Apr;243(16):1640–1643.

16 Levin J. The relationship of proper skin cleansing to pathophysiology, clinical benefits, and the concomitant use of prescription topical therapies in patients with acne vulgaris. *Dermatol Clin.* 2016 Apr;34(2):133–145.

17 Solomon BA, Shalita AR. Effects of detergents on acne. *Clin Dermatol.* 1996 Jan–Feb;14(1):95–99.

18 Nast A, Dréno B, Bettoli V et al; European Dermatology Forum. European evidence-based (S3) guidelines for the treatment of acne. *J Eur Acad Dermatol Venereol*. 2012 Feb;26(Suppl 1):1–29.

19 Bettoli V, Guerra-Tapia A, Herane MI et al. Challenges and solutions in oral isotretinoin in acne: reflections on 35 years of experience. *Clin Cosmet Investig Dermatol*. 2019 Dec;12:943–951.

20 Plewig G, Melnik B, Chen W. *Plewig and Kligman's Acne and Rosaea*. Springer, 2019: fourth edition.

21 British Association of Dermatologists. Patient information leaflet on isotretinoin. Jul 2019. Available from https://www.bad.org. uk/shared/get-file.ashx?id=2314&itemtype=document.

22 Altıntaş Aykan D, Ergün Y. Isotretinoin: still the cause of anxiety for teratogenicity. *Dermatol Ther*. 2020 Jan;33(1):e13192.

23 İslamoğlu ZGK, Altınyazar HC. Effects of isotretinoin on the hair cycle. *J Cosmet Dermatol*. 2019 Apr;18(2):647–651.

24 Karaosmanoğlu N, Mülköğlu C. Analysis of musculoskeletal side effects of oral Isotretinoin treatment: a cross-sectional study. *BMC Musculoskelet Disord*. 2020 Sep;21(1):631.

25 Lee SY, Jamal MM, Nguyen ET et al. Does exposure to isotretinoin increase the risk for the development of inflammatory bowel disease? A meta-analysis. *Eur J Gastroenterol Hepatol*. 2016 Feb; 28(2):210–216.

26 Lee YH, Scharnitz TP, Muscat J et al. Laboratory monitoring during isotretinoin therapy for acne: a systematic review and meta-analysis. *JAMA Dermatol*. 2016 Jan;152(1):35–44.

27 Wootton CI, Cartwright RP, Manning P et al. Should isotretinoin be stopped prior to surgery? A critically appraised topic. *Br J Dermatol*. 2014 Feb;170(2):239–244.

28 Hazen PG, Carney JF, Walker AE et al. Depression – a side effect of 13-cis-retinoic acid therapy. *J Am Acad Dermatol*. 1983;9(2): 278–279.

29 Azoulay L, Blais L, Koren G et al. Isotretinoin and the risk of depression in patients with acne vulgaris: a case-crossover study. *J Clin Psychiatry*. 2008 Apr;69(4):526–532; Bremner JD, Shearer KD, McCaffery PJ. Retinoic acid and affective disorders: the evidence for an association. *J Clin Psychiatry*. 2012 Jan;73(1):37–50.

30 Singer S, Tkachenko E, Sharma P et al. Psychiatric adverse events in patients taking isotretinoin as reported in a Food and Drug Administration database from 1997 to 2017. *JAMA Dermatol*. 2019 Oct;155(10):1162–1166; Kaymak Y, Kalay M, Ilter N et al. Incidence of depression related to isotretinoin treatment in 100 acne vulgaris patients. *Psychol Rep*. 2006;99(3):897–906; Strahan JE, Raimer S. Isotretinoin and the controversy of psychiatric adverse effects. *Int J Dermatol*. 2006;45(7):789–799; Marqueling AL, Zane

LT. Depression and suicidal behavior in acne patients treated with isotretinoin: a systematic review. *Semin Cutan Med Surg.* 2007;26(4): 210–220; Hahm BJ, Min SU, Yoon MY et al. Changes of psychiatric parameters and their relationships by oral isotretinoin in acne patients. *J Dermatol.* 2009;36(5):255–261; Gnanaraj P, Karthikeyan S, Narasimhan M et al. Decrease in 'Hamilton rating scale for depression' following isotretinoin therapy in acne: an open-label prospective study. *Indian J Dermatol.* 2015;60(5):461–464.

31 Hekmatjah J, Chat VS, Sierro TJ et al. Differences in depression and distress between acne patients on isotretinoin vs oral antibiotics. *J Drugs Dermatol.* 2021 Feb;20(2):172–177; Huang YC, Cheng YC. Isotretinoin treatment for acne and risk of depression: A systematic review and meta-analysis. *J Am Acad Dermatol.* 2017 Jun;76(6):1068–1076.e9; Singer S, Tkachenko E, Sharma P et al. Psychiatric adverse events in patients taking isotretinoin as reported in a Food and Drug Administration database from 1997 to 2017. *JAMA Dermatol.* 2019 Oct;155(10):1162–1166.

32 Waldman A, Bolotin D, Arndt KA et al. ASDS guidelines task force: consensus recommendations regarding the safety of lasers, dermabrasion, chemical peels, energy devices, and skin surgery during and after isotretinoin use. *Dermatol Surg.* 2017 Oct;43(10): 1249–1262.

33 Fallah H, Rademaker M. Isotretinoin in the management of acne vulgaris: practical prescribing. *Int J Dermatol.* 2021 Apr;60(4): 451–460.

34 Bagatin E, Costa CS, Rocha MADD et al. Consensus on the use of oral isotretinoin in dermatology – Brazilian Society of Dermatology. *An Bras Dermatol.* 2020 Nov–Dec;95(Suppl 1):19–38.

35 Khanna N, Gupta SD. Acneiform eruptions after facial beauty treatment. *Int J Dermatol.* 1999 Mar;38(3):196–199; Khanna N, Datta Gupta S. Rejuvenating facial massage – a bane or boon? *Int J Dermatol.* 2002 Jul;41(7):407–410.

36 Tan AU, Schlosser BJ, Paller AS. A review of diagnosis and treatment of acne in adult female patients. *Int J Womens Dermatol.* 2017;4(2):56–71.

37 Griffiths WA. The red face – an overview and delineation of the MARSH syndrome. *Clin Exp Dermatol.* 1999 Jan;24(1):42–47.

38 Kligman AM. An overview of acne. *J Invest Dermatol.* 1974 Mar;62(3):268–287.

39 Chen Y, Lyga J. Brain-skin connection: stress, inflammation and skin aging. *Inflamm Allergy Drug Targets.* 2014;13(3):177–190.

40 Plewig G, Melnik B, Chen W. *Plewig and Kligman's Acne and Rosaea.* Springer, 2019: fourth edition.

41 Rubenstein RM, Malerich SA. Malassezia (pityrosporum) folliculitis. *J Clin Aesthet Dermatol.* 2014 Mar;7(3):37–41.

42 Ibid.

43 Seneschal J, Kubica E, Boursault L et al. Exogenous inflammatory acne due to combined application of cosmetic and facial rubbing. *Dermatology*. 2012;224(3):221–223.

44 Fulton JE Jr, Pay SR, Fulton JE 3rd. Comedogenicity of current therapeutic products, cosmetics, and ingredients in the rabbit ear. *J Am Acad Dermatol*. 1984 Jan;10(1):96–105; Kligman AM, Mills OH Jr. 'Acne cosmetica'. *Arch Dermatol*. 1972 Dec;106(6): 843–850.

45 Basler RS. Acne mechanica in athletes. *Cutis*. 1992 Aug;50(2): 125–128; Mills OH Jr, Kligman A. Acne mechanica. *Arch Dermatol*. 1975 Apr;111(4):481–483.

46 Khanna N, Datta Gupta S. Rejuvenating facial massage – a bane or boon? *Int J Dermatol*. 2002 Jul;41(7):407–410.

47 Vongraviopap S, Asawanonda P. Dark chocolate exacerbates acne. *Int J Dermatol*. 2016 May;55(5):587–591.

48 Delost GR, Delost ME, Lloyd J. The impact of chocolate consumption on acne vulgaris in college students: a randomized crossover study. *J Am Acad Dermatol*. 2016 Jul;75(1):220–222.

49 LaRosa CL, Quach KA, Koons K et al. Consumption of dairy in teenagers with and without acne. *J Am Acad Dermatol*. 2016 Aug;75(2):318–22.

50 Berra B, Rizzo AM. Glycemic index, glycemic load: new evidence for a link with acne. *J Am Coll Nutr*. 2009 Aug;28(Suppl): 450S–454S.

51 Lee SJ, Seok J, Jeong SY et al. Facial pores: definition, causes, and treatment options. *Dermatol Surg*. 2016 Mar;42(3):277–285.

52 Jung HJ, Ahn JY, Lee JI et al. Analysis of the number of enlarged pores according to site, age, and sex. *Skin Res Technol*. 2018 Aug;24(3):367–370.

53 Sakuma TH, Maibach HI. Oily skin: an overview. *Skin Pharmacol Physiol*. 2012;25(5):227–235.

54 Shuo L, Ting Y, KeLun W et al. Efficacy and possible mechanisms of botulinum toxin treatment of oily skin. *J Cosmet Dermatol*. 2019 Apr;18(2):451–457.

55 Singh Y, Neema S, Bahuguna A et al. Sebaceous filaments. *Dermatol Pract Concept*. 2021 Jan;11(1):e2021148.

56 Ibid.

Chapter 13: Rosacea

1 Gether L, Overgaard LK, Egeberg A et al. Incidence and prevalence of rosacea: a systematic review and meta analysis. *Br J Dermatol*. 2018 Aug;179(2):282–289.

2 Plewig G, Melnik B, Chen W. *Plewig and Kligman's Acne and Rosaea*. Springer, 2019: fourth edition.

3 Marks R. The enigma of rosacea. *J Dermatolog Treat*. 2007;18(6): 326–328.

4 Plewig G, Melnik B, Chen W. *Plewig and Kligman's Acne and Rosaea*. Springer, 2019: fourth edition.

5 Ibid.

6 Marks R. The enigma of rosacea. *J Dermatolog Treat*. 2007;18(6): 326–328.

7 Kyriakou G, Glentis A. Skin in the game: video-game-related cutaneous pathologies in adolescents. *Int J Pediatr Adolesc Med*. 2021 Jun;8(2):68–75.

8 Schaller M, Almeida LMC, Bewley A et al. Recommendations for rosacea diagnosis, classification, and management: update from the global ROSacea COnsensus 2019 panel. *Br J Dermatol*. 2020 May;182(5):1269–1276.

9 Ibid.

10 Ertl GA, Levine N, Kligman AM. A comparison of the efficacy of topical tretinoin and low-dose oral isotretinoin in rosacea. *Arch Dermatol*. 1994;130(3):319–324.

11 Plewig G, Melnik B, Chen W. *Plewig and Kligman's Acne and Rosaea*. Springer, 2019: fourth edition.

12 Ibid; Zhang H, Tang K, Wang Y et al. Use of botulinum toxin in treating rosacea: a systematic review. *Clin Cosmet Investig Dermatol*. 2021 Apr;14:407–417.

13 Ozbagcivan O, Akarsu S, Dolas N et al. Contact sensitization to cosmetic series of allergens in patients with rosacea: a prospective controlled study. *J Cosmet Dermatol*. 2020;19:173–179.

14 Plewig G, Melnik B, Chen W. *Plewig and Kligman's Acne and Rosaea*. Springer, 2019: fourth edition.

15 Hanna E, Xing L, Taylor JH et al. Role of botulinum toxin A in improving facial erythema and skin quality. *Arch Dermatol Res*. 2021 Sep;14.

16 Oh YJ, Lee NY, Suh DH et al. A split-face study using botulinum toxin type B to decrease facial erythema index. *J Cosmet Laser Ther*. 2011 Oct;13(5):243–248; Kim MJ, Kim JH, Cheon HI et al. Assessment of skin physiology change and safety after intradermal injections with botulinum toxin: a randomized, double-blind, placebo-controlled, split-face pilot study in rosacea patients with facial erythema. *Dermatol Surg*. 2019 Sep;45(9):1155–1162.

17 Al-Niaimi F, Glagoleva E, Araviiskaia E. Pulsed dye laser followed by intradermal botulinum toxin type-A in the treatment of rosacea-associated erythema and flushing. *Dermatol Ther*. 2020 Nov;33(6):e13976.

18 Friedman O, Koren A, Niv R et al. The toxic edge – a novel treatment for refractory erythema and flushing of rosacea. *Lasers Surg Med.* 2019 Apr;51(4):325–331.

19 Zhang H, Tang K, Wang Y et al. Use of botulinum toxin in treating rosacea: a systematic review. *Clin Cosmet Investig Dermatol.* 2021 Apr;14:407–417.

20 Seo BH, Kim DH, Suh HS et al. Facial flushing and erythema of rosacea improved by carvedilol. *Dermatol Ther.* 2020 Nov;33(6):e14520; Hsu CC, Lee JY. Carvedilol for the treatment of refractory facial flushing and persistent erythema of rosacea. *Arch Dermatol.* 2011 Nov;147(11):1258–1260.

21 James WDI, Elston DM, Treat J et al. *Andrews' Diseases of the Skin: Clinical Dermatology.* Elsevier, 2020: thirteenth edition.

22 Mekić S, Hamer MA, Wigmann C et al. Epidemiology and determinants of facial telangiectasia: a cross-sectional study. *J Eur Acad Dermatol Venereol.* 2020 Apr;34(4):821–826.

23 Zhang H, Tang K, Wang Y et al. Use of botulinum toxin in treating rosacea: a systematic review. *Clin Cosmet Investig Dermatol.* 2021 Apr;14:407–417.

24 Liapakis I, Englander M, Sinani R et al. Management of facial telangiectasias with hand cautery. *World J Plast Surg.* 2015 Jul;4(2): 127–133.

Chapter 14: Dermatitis

1 Tolaymat L, Hall MR. Perioral dermatitis. *StatPearls* [Internet]. 2021 Sep.

2 Tempark T, Shwayder TA. Perioral dermatitis: a review of the condition with special attention to treatment options. *Am J Clin Dermatol.* 2014 Apr;15(2):101–113.

3 Dessinioti C, Katsambas A. Seborrheic dermatitis: etiology, risk factors, and treatments: facts and controversies. *Clin Dermatol.* 2013 Jul–Aug;31(4):343–351.

4 Rebora A, Rongioletti F. The red face: seborrheic dermatitis. *Clin Dermatol.* 1993 Apr–Jun;11(2):243–251.

5 Zirwas MJ. Contact dermatitis to cosmetics. *Clin Rev Allergy Immunol.* 2019 Feb;56(1):119–128.

6 Ibid.

7 Castanedo-Tardan MP, Zug KA. Patterns of cosmetic contact allergy. *Dermatol Clin.* 2009 Jul;27(3):265–280, vi.

8 Park ME, Zippin JH. Allergic contact dermatitis to cosmetics. *Dermatol Clin.* 2014 Jan;32(1):1–11.

Chapter 15: Melasma and Facial Hyperpigmentation

1   Spierings, NMK. Melasma: A critical analysis of clinical trials investigating treatment modalities published in the past 10 years. *J Cosmetic Dermatol.* 2020 Jun;19(6):1284–1289.

2   Griffiths CEM, Kang S, Ellis CN et al. Two concentrations of topical tretinoin (retinoic acid) cause similar improvement of photoaging but different degree of irritation. *Arch Dermatol.* 1995;131:1037–1044; Renova (tretinoin cream) leaflet. Available from https://www.accessdata.fda.gov/drugsatfda_docs/label/2014/021108s015lbl.pdf.

3   Rendon MI, Benitez AL, Gaviria JI. Telangiectatic melasma: a new entity? *Cosmetic Derm.* 2007 Mar;20(3):144–149.

4   Kligman AM, Willis I. A new formula for depigmenting human skin. *Arch Dermatol.* 1975;111:40–48.

5   Bhawan J, Grimes P, Pandya AG et al. A histological examination for skin atrophy after 6 months of treatment with fluocinolone acetonide 0.01%, hydroquinone 4%, and tretinoin 0.05% cream. *Am J Dermatopathol.* 2009 Dec;31(8):794–798.

6   Sanchez NP, Pathak MA, Sato S et al. Melasma: a clinical, light microscopic, ultrastructural, and immunofluorescence study. *J Am Acad Dermatol.* 1981 Jun;4(6):698–710.

7   Kang WH, Yoon KH, Lee ES et al. Melasma: histopathological characteristics in 56 Korean patients. *Br J Dermatol.* 2002 Feb;146(2):228–237.

8   Spierings, NMK. Melasma: A critical analysis of clinical trials investigating treatment modalities published in the past 10 years. *J Cosmetic Dermatol.* 2020 Jun;19(6):1284–1289.

9   Rajanala S, Maymone MBC, Vashi NA. Melasma pathogenesis: a review of the latest research, pathological findings, and investigational therapies. *Dermatol Online J.* 2019 Oct;25(10):13030/qt47b7r28c; Lee AY. Recent progress in melasma pathogenesis. *Pigment Cell Melanoma Res.* 2015 Nov;28(6):648–660.

10 Nijor T. Treatment of melasma with tranexamic acid. *Clin Res.* 1979;13:3129–3131.

11 Maeda K, Tomita Y. Mechanism of the inhibitory effect of tranexamic acid on melanogenesis in cultured human melanocytes in the presence of keratinocyte-conditioned medium. *J Health Sci.* 2007;53:389–396.

12 Padhi T, Pradhan S. Oral tranexamic acid with fluocinolone-based triple combination cream versus fluocinolone-based triple combination cream alone in melasma: an open labeled randomized comparative trial. *Indian J Dermatol.* 2015 Sep–Oct;60(5):520; Karn D, Kc S, Amatya A et al. Oral tranexamic acid for the

treatment of melasma. *Kathmandu Univ Med J (KUMJ)*. 2012 Oct–Dec;10(40):40–43.

13 Mansouri P, Farshi S, Hashemi Z et al. Evaluation of the efficacy of cysteamine 5% cream in the treatment of epidermal melasma: a randomized double-blind placebo-controlled trial. *Br J Dermatol*. 2015 Jul;173(1):209–217; Farshi S, Mansouri P, Kasraee B. Efficacy of cysteamine cream in the treatment of epidermal melasma, evaluating by Dermacatch as a new measurement method: a randomized double blind placebo controlled study. *J Dermatolog Treat*. 2018 Mar;29(2):182–189.

Part 5: How to Tackle Common Aesthetic Concerns

1 Balin AK, Kligman AM (eds). *Aging and the Skin*. Raven Press, 1989.

Chapter 16: Fine Lines and Wrinkles

1 Manríquez JJ, Cataldo K, Vera-Kellet C et al. Wrinkles. *BMJ Clin Evid*. 2014 Dec;2014:1711.

2 Ibid.

3 Ibid.

4 Ibid.

5 Schantz EJ, Johnson EA. Botulinum toxin: the story of its development for the treatment of human disease. *Perspect Biol Med*. 1997;40:317–327; Albanese A. Discussion of unique properties of botulinum toxins. *Toxicon*. 2009;54:702–708.

6 Norman S. Lifting effect of onabotulinumtoxinA in patients treated for glabellar and crow's feet rhytids. *J Cosmet Laser Ther*. 2020 Nov;22(6–8):232–238.

7 Albrecht P, Jansen A, Lee JI et al. High prevalence of neutralizing antibodies after long-term botulinum neurotoxin therapy. *Neurology*. 2019 Jan;92(1):e48–e54; Fabbri M, Leodori G, Fernandes RM et al. Neutralizing antibody and botulinum toxin therapy: a systematic review and meta-analysis. *Neurotox Res*. 2016 Jan;29(1):105–117.

8 Binder WJ. Long-term effects of botulinum toxin type A (Botox) on facial lines: a comparison in identical twins. *Arch Facial Plast Surg*. 2006 Nov–Dec;8(6):426–431; Rivkin A, Binder WJ. Long-term effects of onabotulinumtoxinA on facial lines: a 19-year experience of identical twins. *Dermatol Surg*. 2015 Jan;41(Suppl 1):S64–S66.

9   Humphrey S. Neurotoxins: evidence for prevention. *J Drugs Dermatol*. 2017 Jun;16(6):s87–s90.

Chapter 17: Dark Under-Eye Circles

1   Nayak CS, Giri AS, Zambare US. A study of clinicopathological correlation of periorbital hyperpigmentation. *Indian Dermatol Online J*. 2018 Jul–Aug;9(4):245–249.

2   Ibid.

3   Mendiratta V, Rana S, Jassi R et al. Study of causative factors and clinical patterns of periorbital pigmentation. *Indian Dermatol Online J*. 2019 May–Jun;10(3):293–295.

4   Ibid.

5   Friedmann DP, Goldman MP. Dark circles: etiology and management options. *Clin Plast Surg*. 2015 Jan;42(1):33–50.

6   Vrcek I, Ozgur O, Nakra T. Infraorbital dark circles: a review of the pathogenesis, evaluation and treatment. *J Cutan Aesthet Surg*. 2016 Apr–Jun;9(2):65–72.

7   NHS. The eatwell guide. 28 Jan 2019. Available from https://www.nhs.uk/live-well/eat-well/the-eatwell-guide.

8   Roh MR, Chung KY. Infraorbital dark circles: definition, causes, and treatment options. *Dermatol Surg*. 2009 Aug;35(8):1163–1171.

Chapter 18: Unwanted or Excess Facial Hair

1   Richards RN, Meharg GE. Electrolysis: observations from 13 years and 140,000 hours of experience. *J Am Acad Dermatol*. 1995 Oct;33(4):662–666.

2   Alijanpour R, Aliakbarpour F. A randomized clinical trial on the comparison between hair shaving and snipping prior to laser hair removal sessions in women suffering from hirsutism. *J Cosmet Dermatol*. 2017 Mar;16(1):70–75.

3   Lizneva D, Gavrilova-Jordan L, Walker W et al. Androgen excess: investigations and management. *Best Pract Res Clin Obstet Gynaecol*. 2016 Nov;37:98–118.

4   Dawber RP. Guidance for the management of hirsutism. *Curr Med Res Opin*. 2005 Aug;21(8):1227–1234.

5   Snast I, Kaftory R, Lapidoth M et al. Paradoxical hypertrichosis associated with laser and light therapy for hair removal: a systematic review and meta-analysis. *Am J Clin Dermatol*. 2021 Sep;22(5):615–624.

6   Ibid.

7   Alijanpour R, Aliakbarpour F. A randomized clinical trial on the comparison between hair shaving and snipping prior to laser hair removal sessions in women suffering from hirsutism. *J Cosmet Dermatol*. 2017 Mar;16(1):70–75.

8   Olsen EA. Methods of hair removal. *J Am Acad Dermatol*. 1999 Feb;40(2 Pt 1):143–155; quiz:156–157.

9   Dorgham NA, Dorgham DA. Lasers for reduction of unwanted hair in skin of colour: a systematic review and meta-analysis. *J Eur Acad Dermatol Venereol*. 2020 May;34(5):948–955.

10 Richards RN, Meharg GE. Electrolysis: observations from 13 years and 140,000 hours of experience. *J Am Acad Dermatol*. 1995 Oct;33(4):662–666.

11 Ibid.

12 Shapiro J, Lui H. Vaniqa--eflornithine 13.9% cream. *Skin Therapy Lett*. 2001 Apr;6(7):1–3, 5.

13 Shenenberger DW, Utecht LM. Removal of unwanted facial hair. *Am Fam Physician*. 2002 Nov;66(10):1907–1911.

14 Olsen EA. Methods of hair removal. *J Am Acad Dermatol*. 1999 Feb;40(2 Pt 1):143–155; quiz:156–157; Lynfield YL, Macwilliams P. Shaving and hair growth. *J Invest Dermatol*. 1970 Sep;55(3): 170–172.

15 Fezza JP, Klippenstein KA, Wesley RE. Cilia regrowth of shaven eyebrows. *Arch Facial Plast Surg*. 1999 Jul–Sep;1(3):223–224.

16 Flaharty PM, Flaharty KK, Gorman L. Latisse (bimatoprost) for enhancement of eyelashes. *Insight*. 2014 summer;39(3):24–26.

17 Filippopoulos T, Paula JS, Torun N et al. Periorbital changes associated with topical bimatoprost. *Ophthalmic Plast Reconstr Surg*. 2008 Jul–Aug;24(4):302–307.

18 Jayaprakasam A, Ghazi-Nouri S. Periorbital fat atrophy – an unfamiliar side effect of prostaglandin analogues. *Orbit*. 2010 Dec;29(6):357–359.

19 Vergilis-Kalner IJ. Application of bimatoprost ophthalmic solution 0.03% for the treatment of eyebrow hypotrichosis: series of ten cases. *Dermatol Online J*. 2014 Jun;20(6):13030/qt1mc5v5mx.

Chapter 19: Skin 'Rejuvenation'

1   Khanna N, Datta Gupta S. Rejuvenating facial massage – a bane or boon? *Int J Dermatol*. 2002 Jul;41(7):407–410.

2   Khanna N, Gupta SD. Acneiform eruptions after facial beauty treatment. *Int J Dermatol*. 1999 Mar;38(3):196–199.

3   Handler MZ, Goldberg DJ. Neocollagenesis. In: Goldberg DJ (ed). *Dermal Fillers*. Karger Publishers, 2018;vol. 4:27–35.

4 Honeybrook A, Bernstein E. Oral isotretinoin and photoaging: a review. *J Cosmet Dermatol*. 2020 Jul;19(7):1548–1554.

5 Kligman LH. Photoaging. Manifestations, prevention, and treatment. *Dermatol Clin*. 1986 Jul;4(3):517–528.

6 Handler MZ, Goldberg DJ. Neocollagenesis. In: Goldberg DJ (ed). *Dermal Fillers*. Karger Publishers, 2018;vol. 4:27–35.

7 Ibid.

8 Goldberg D, Guana A, Volk A et al. Single-arm study for the characterization of human tissue response to injectable poly-L-lactic acid. *Dermatol Surg*. 2013 Jun;39(6):915–922.

9 Emer J, Sundaram H. Aesthetic applications of calcium hydroxylapatite volumizing filler: an evidence-based review and discussion of current concepts: (part 1 of 2). *J Drugs Dermatol*. 2013 Dec;12(12): 1345–1354.

10 Karnik J, Baumann L, Bruce S et al. A double-blind, randomized, multicenter, controlled trial of suspended polymethylmethacrylate microspheres for the correction of atrophic facial acne scars. *J Am Acad Dermatol*. 2014 Jul;71(1):77–83.

11 Kim JA, Van Abel D. Neocollagenesis in human tissue injected with a polycaprolactone-based dermal filler. *J Cosmet Laser Ther*. 2015 Apr;17(2):99–101.

12 Kerscher M, Bayrhammer J, Reuther T. Rejuvenating influence of a stabilized hyaluronic acid-based gel of nonanimal origin on facial skin aging. *Dermatol Surg*. 2008 May;34(5):720–726.

13 Narins DJ, Narins RS. Non-surgical radiofrequency facelift. *J Drugs Dermatol*. 2003 Oct;2(5):495–500; Gold MH. Tissue tightening: a hot topic utilizing deep dermal heating. *J Drugs Dermatol*. 2007 Dec;6(12):1238–1242; Abraham MT, Chiang SK, Keller GS et al. Clinical evaluation of non-ablative radiofrequency facial rejuvenation. *J Cosmet Laser Ther*. 2004 Nov;6(3):136–144; Prendergast PM. Augmentation with injectable fillers. In: *Aesthetic Medicine*. Springer, 2012: 297–335.

14 Alam M, White LE, Martin N et al. Ultrasound tightening of facial and neck skin: a rater-blinded prospective cohort study. *J Am Acad Dermatol*. 2010 Feb;62(2):262–269.

15 Gülbitti HA, Colebunders B, Pirayesh A et al. Thread-lift sutures: still in the lift? A systematic review of the literature. *Plas Recon Surg*. 2018 Mar;141(3):341e–347e.

16 Kaminer MS, Bogart M, Choi C et al. Long-term efficacy of anchored barbed sutures in the face and neck. *Dermatol Surg*. 2008;34:1041–1047; de Benito J, Pizzamiglio R, Theodorou D et al. Facial rejuvenation and improvement of malar projection using sutures with absorbable cones: Surgical technique and case series. *Aesthetic Plast Surg*. 2011;35:248–253.

17 Aust MC, Reimers K, Gohritz A et al. Percutaneous collagen induction. Scarless skin rejuvenation: fact or fiction? *Clin Exp Dermatol.* 2010 Jun;35(4):437–439.

18 Alster TS, Graham PM. Microneedling: a review and practical guide. *Dermatol Surg.* 2018 Mar;44(3):397–404.

19 Ibid.

Index

Page references in *italics* indicate images.

acetylcholine (ACH) 208, 209, 234–5, 240

acid mantle 17

acids 147–52

acne: acne cosmetica 64, 65, 67, 196; acneiform 194–5, 260, 261; acne mechanica 196 acne vulgaris 9, 29, 30–1, 35, 64, 66–7, 106, 150, 151, 156, 161, 163–200, 201, 202, 215, 246, 253; adult women and 189–93; atrophic acne scars 193–4, 265; bacteria 165; chocolate and 196–8; enlarged pores 198–9; exogeneous acne 195–6; follicular hyperkeratinisation 164; 'fungal' 194–5; hormonal stimulation of sebaceous galands 164; inflammation 165–6; 'mild' acne 163–4; 'popping' a pimple 167–8; pregnancy and breastfeeding and 193; sebaceous filaments 200; stages of an acne lesion *166*; teenagers and 187–9; treatments 168–87

adapalene 122, 170–2, 174

adenosine triphosphate (ATP) 142

adjunctive therapy 177–9

aesthetic concerns, common 231–72

ageing 9, 28, 31, 45, 60, 79, 81, 87, 90, 95, 96, 103, 104, 105, 106, 107, 109, 122, 123, 128, 129, 130, 143, 145, 154, 155, 199, 211, 223, 231, 233, 240, 274; butt skin test 48–9; collagen and 52–6, *53, 55*; elastin 56; epidermis 49–51; extrinsic 47–8; facial skin sagging 57; intrinsic 47–9, 223; skin changes and 47–58, *53, 58*; topical tretinoin and 206; vitamin A and 124–7

Aging and the Skin (Balin/Kligman) 11, 231

Alexandrite laser 248, 251

alpha-hydroxy acids 147–9, 193

amino acids 104, 133, 228

androgen hormones 30, 64, 164, 175, 189–91, 193, 199, 245–8

antibiotics 107, 168, 171, 182, 188, 207; oral 173–4, 176, 178, 185, 193, 194, 195, 216; resistance 174

antioxidants 37, 60, 142–4, 183

Ardena Skin Tonic 60

Arden, Elizabeth 60

astringents 97

atopic dermatitis (eczema) 16, 20, 39, 67, 78, 218

azelaic acid 107, 116, 150–1, 168, 177, 193, 206–7

bakuchiol 116, 154–6
basal cells/basal keratinocytes 21–3, 26, 50
benzoyl peroxide 73, 168, 172, 174, 176–7, 178, 188, 193
Big Skincare 1, 5, 6–7, 8, 9, 13, 14, 16, 17, 19, 21, 25, 26, 27, 28, 29, 33, 42, 47, 52, 57, 61, 64, 67, 68, 70, 71, 81, 87, 96, 98, 101, 102, 107; bakuchiol and 154, 155; HA creams and 152; ingredient claims 111–58; melasma and 221; skin rejuvenation treatments and 259; vitamin C and 145
biostimulators 265, 269
blackheads 176, 178, 198, 200
blue light 95, 96, 172
botulinum toxin 106, 199, 234–40, 246; forehead acne and 240; immunity 239; questions 237–40
butt skin test 48–9

calcium hydroxylapatite (CaHa) 265
cancer 2, 24, 34, 48, 87, 90, 91, 96, 108, 130, 135, 136, 137, 143, 231
carvedilol 209–10
ceramides 19, 20, 21, 32, 51
Chanel Precision Ultra Correction Restructuring Anti-Wrinkle Firming Cream SPF 10 81
chocolate, acne and 196–8
cholesterol 19, 51, 141, 181, 184–5
coconut oil 69, 82
coenzyme Q10 37
collagen 7, 153, 154, 193, 203, 244, 274; ageing of skin and 47, 49, 52–6, 55; skin rejuvenation and 259, 260, 262, 263, 264, 265, 266,

267–8, 270–1; skin structure and 21, 26, 27, 28, 31; supplement 104–5; vitamins and 123, 124, 129, 141, 144, 145
comedogenicity 63–7, 77, 196, 261
comedones 64–6, 77, 122, 130, 150, 163, 165–6, 170, 178, 181, 188, 196, 201, 215, 260, 261
compounded skincare 148–9
contraceptive pill 175
copper peptides 153–4, 176, 183, 188, 199, 221, 247
corneocytes 15–17, 18, 19, 22, 32, 34, 41, 42, 51, 78, 99, 114, 148, 183, 200
corneodesmosomes 15, 18
cosmeceutical 106–7, 111
Créme Valaze 59–60
cutaneous reaction pattern 40
cyclopentasiloxane 73
cysteamine cream 228–9
cytokines 18–19

darker skin 48, 91, 201, 212, 251
dark under-eye circles 9, 241–4
depression 161, 185, 243
'dermal' melasma 225–9
dermal papilla 30, 252
dermaplaning 253–5
dermatitis 16, 20, 39, 51, 67, 78, 82, 128–9, 161, 169, 204–5, 215–20, 261, 271; facial or eyelid eczema 218–20; perioral dermatitis 215–16; seborrheic dermatitis 216–17
dermatologist, choosing 277–8
dermis 116, 117, 153–4, 254; acne and 193, 199; ageing of 47–8, 49, 50, 52–6, 53, 55, 57; dark circles and 241, 244; hydroquinone and 135;

melasma 223, 224, 225; rejuvenation 259, 260, 263, 264, 265–6, 267, 270, 271, 272; rosacea and 202, 203, 208–9, 210; skin type and 34, 44; structure of skin and 12, 19, 21, 25, 26–7, 28, 29, 31, *31*; vitamin A and 122, 123, 129; vitamin C and 144, 145

desquamation 15, 40

Dianette 175

dihydrotestosterone 164, 247

dimethicone 72, 73, 98

diode laser 251

double cleansing 70

dry skin 38–42, 67, 68, 71, 72, 89, 99, 128, 179, 205, 207, 218

eczema 20, 39, 67, 74, 78–9, 108, 149, 158, 227, 242; facial 218–20

eflornithine cream 252–3

elastin 21, 27, 47, 48, 49, 56, 57, 144, 145, 153, 154, 193, 203, 210–11, 260, 263, 265

electrolysis 132, 186, 248, 251–2

endoplasmic reticulum (ER) 202

energy-based treatments 266–7

epidermis *31*, 32, 44, 47, 48, 98–9, 116, 122, 123, 124, 131, 133, 144, 152, 169, 219, 224, 225, 249–50, 263, 270, 271; ageing and 49–51; viable epidermis 21–6, 78

evidence-based skincare 4, 5–6, 8–9

exfoliating 1, 16, 98–9, 100, 123, 131–2, 148, 158, 178; 'regular exfoliation' 15

exogeneous acne 195–6

exogeneous ochronosis 135–6

extrinsic ageing 47–8

eye cream 1, 2, 7, 98, 101, 109, 125, 158, 244

eyelash and eyebrow hypotrichosis (thin/short eyelashes) 255–7

facelifts, 'non-surgical' 267–8

face masks 102–3

face wipe 68, 69

facial hair 9, 132, 192, 245–57; darker skin and 251; dermaplaning and 253–5; eflornithine cream and 252–3; electrolysis and 251–2; eyelash and eyebrow hypotrichosis (thin/short eyelashes) 255–6; hair removal 248–51; hair types 245; idiopathic hirsutism 245–6; lasers and intense pulsed light (IPL) 248–9; Latisse 256; periorbital fat atrophy 256; snipping hair between laser or IPL treatments 249–50

facial or eyelid eczema 218–20

facials 2, 25, 170, 182, 188, 260–1

facial sagging 57–8

facial yoga 105–6

fatty acids 19, 68, 142, 173

FDA (US Food and Drug Administration) 63–4, 93, 106, 113, 122, 123, 124, 125, 135, 175, 208, 224, 233, 250, 253, 266, 268

fibroblast 28, *31*, 54–5, *55*, 56, 124, 135, 264, 265

fillers 264–6

fine lines 14, 73, 87, 102, 111, 123, 125, 126, 130, 131, 132, 155, 233, 253, 259, 262, 266, 270, 274, 275; 500 dalton rule 115–16

flaky skin 40, 128, 215

flannels 69

follicular hyperkeratinisation 164

free radicals 87, 96, 142–3
'fungal' acne 194–5

glycerol 68, 78
glycolic acid 99, 108, 116, 147–8, 217, 221, 226
glycoproteins 27
glycosaminoglycans 27
granular phase 22
ground substance 27

hair follicles 8, 29, 30–1, 34, 36, 63, 64, 65, 67, 114, 115, 122, 123, 164, 166–7, 168, 170, 172, 173, 177, 178, 180, 184, 189, 194–5, 196, 197, 198, 199, 200, 202, 240, 246–7, 248, 250, 252
hand cautery (electrosurgery) 211, 212–13
high-frequency ultrasound (HIFU) 267–9
HMG-CoA reductase 51
hormone replacement therapy (HRT) 262, 272
humectant 18, 32, 41, 42, 72, 79, 102
hyaluronic acid (HA) 27–8, 102, 116, 151–2, 243, 264
hydroquinone 107, 116, 133–40, 148, 151, 222, 224, 225, 228, 229, 274; cancer and 136; cycles of 137–8; exogeneous ochronosis and 135–6; melasma and facial hyperpigmentation, treating with 138–9; questions 136–8; rebound pigmentation and 136; safety 134–6
hyperpigmentation 133, 136, 138, 251, 274; facial 221–9

ichthyosis 16, 99
idiopathic hirsutism 246–8

in-office: cosmetic procedures 226, 266, 269, 272; sale of cosmetic skincare products 157–8
inflammation 19, 43, 48, 51, 74; acne and 165–6, 168, 169, 171, 173, 174, 175, 176, 178, 180, 182, 183, 193, 194, 196, 197; azelaic acid and 150, 151; dark under-eye circles and 242; dermatitis and 217, 218, 220; melasma and 224, 227; niacinamide and 156; petroleum jelly and 75; post-inflammatory hyperpigmentation 133; rosacea and 202, 206–7; vitamin C and 143
injectable hydrators 265–6
intense pulsed light (IPL) 212, 248–51, 266
intrinsic ageing 47–9, 223
isotretinoin 176–7, 179–87, 190, 199, 200, 203, 207, 252, 262–3

jade face roller 101–2

keratin 15, 18, 22, 32, 164, 166, 167, 200, 240, 254; keratinocytes 21–4, 32, 50–1, 99, 123, 124, 134, 177, 180, 197, 224, 228; keratinisation 32, 164, 180, 240
Kligman, Dr Albert 74, 75, 76–7, 106–7, 112, 126, 190, 231, 279
Koebner phenomenon 75
Korean skincare 100–1

lasers 38, 132, 170, 208, 211–12, 226, 266; ablative resurfacing 194, 199, 270; CO_2 233, 267; facial 127; hair removal 186, 248–51,

254; Nd:YAG 212, 248, 251;
peel 75; pulsed dye 209
Latisse 255–6
lauric acid 82
LED masks 103–4, 157
light therapies 172–3
lipid bilayer 19–20, 115
lipid matrix 17, 19, 51, 78

Malassezia 194, 195, 217
matrix metalloproteinases
(MMPs) 52–6
mechanical cleansing devices
99–100
melanin 23, 24, 25, 133, *134*, 138,
212, 224, 225, 226, 241, 248
melanocyte 23–5, 133, *134*, 135,
138, 225, 228
melanosomes 23–4, 25
melasma 9, 108, 133, 135, 136,
137, 138–9, 148, 150, 151,
158, 182, 221–9, 231, 273–4;
cysteamine cream and
228–9; 'dermal' melasma
225; heat and 226–7; peels
to treat 226; steroids in
treatment for 224;
tranexamic acid (TXA)
tablets and 227–8;
treatments 222–3; triple
combination and
telangiectasia 223–4
MHRA (Medicines and
Healthcare Products
Regulatory Agency) 113,
224, 252–3
microdermabrasion 25, 99, 170,
196
microneedling 25, 127, 266–7,
270–2
modern skincare, origins of
59–61
moisturiser 1, 2, 7, 9, 11, 20–1, 41,
44, 49, 61, 63, 65, 70–85, 87,
98, 99, 101, 102, 107, 108,

116, 125, 127, 132, 153, 154,
155, 156, 158, 177, 182, 208,
220, 221, 274, 276; acne and
179; brands 79–82; coconut
oil 82; 'normal' skin 77–8;
origins of 70–1; private-label
companies 82–5; silicones
73; skin diseases and 78–9;
types 72; Vaseline/
petroleum jelly 74–7
mucocutaneous side effects
183–4
naevi 25
natural moisturising factors
(NMFs) 16, 32, 41, 42
'natural' skincare 100
neocollagenesis 54, 260, 264,
265
neurotoxin 106, 208–9, 234, 240
niacinamide 108, 116, 156, 221

oestrogens 175, 190, 199, 247,
262
oily skin 1, 29, 34–7, 38, 39, 97,
189, 195, 200, 275

papillary dermis 21
period spots 190–2
perioral dermatitis 161, 215–16,
271
petrolatum 72, 73, 74, 76, 77, 78,
156
petroleum jelly 64, 71, 74, 75–7
pigmentation 14, 23, 25, 48, 108,
231, 251, 256, 274, 275;
hydroquinone and 130, 133,
134, 135–9, 145; melasma
and facial 221–9;
niacinamide and 156;
pigment-correcting cosmetic
skincare products 25
plaque psoriasis 75
polycystic ovary syndrome
(PCOS) 192, 245–7
poly-L-lactic acid (PLLA) 265

polymethylmethacrylate (PMMA) 265

pores, skin 48, 63–4, 73, 101, 114, 145, 165, 173; blackhead and 200; enlarged 48, 145, 198–9; petroleum jelly and 76–7; pore-clogging products 64, 65

positive controls 64, 65

post-inflammatory hyperpigmentation (PIH) 133, 251

private-label companies 82–5

Procter and Gamble 70–1

prolyl hydroxylase 28

psoriasis 22, 75, 122, 217

rabbit ear model 64

regenerating products 23, 274

Renova 122, 124

reticular dermis 21

retinoic acid 116, 121–6, 128, 154, 169, 171, 180, 223, 252, 263, 274

retinoids 73, 100, 121–2, 128–32, 168, 169, 176, 177, 179, 181, 188, 233, 244; purge 170–1; questions about 128–31; retinoid dermatitis 128–9, 169; skincare products, how to use with other 131–2; topical 100, 128–31, 169, 170, 171, 176, 181, 188, 233, 244

retinol 121, 124, 125, 126, 154, 155

rosacea 67, 150, 156, 158, 161, 201–13, 223–4, 252, 254, 271, 273; carvedilol 209–10; causes 202–4; flushing and redness, treatments of 207–10; hand cautery 212–13; lasers 211–12; neurotoxin 208–9; papules and pustules, topical treatments for treatment of 206–7; screen dermatitis 204–5; telangiectasia 210–13; topical tretinoin for anti-ageing 206

routine, building skincare 158

salicylic acid (SA) 106, 116, 149–50, 168, 217

scars 54, 161, 166, 167, 169, 180, 189; atrophic acne 193–4, 265, 270; collagen and 54; dermaplaning and 253; electrolysis 252; surgery and 278

screen dermatitis 204–5

sebaceous filaments 9, 200

sebaceous glands 29–30, 31, 34, 35–6, 37, 41, 164, 166, 167, 173, 180, 184, 191, 193, 195, 197, 203, 205

sebaceous hyperplasia 35, 38

sebocytes 29–30, 180, 209

seborrheic dermatitis 216–17, 219

sensitive (reactive) skin 42–4, 205, 206, 207

serum 2, 7, 11, 16, 49, 61, 72, 102, 109, 111, 125, 132, 142, 156, 158, 221

silicones 73

skincare influencers ('skinfluencer') 7, 8, 70, 159, 274

skincare products you don't need 97–109; collagen/skin supplements 104–5; cosmeceuticals/medical-grade skincare 106–9; exfoliants/scrubs 98–9; eye cream 98; face masks 102–3; face yoga 105–6; jade rollers 101–2; Korean skincare 100–1; LED masks 103–4; mechanical cleansing devices 99–100;

natural skincare 100;
serums 102; toner 97
skin colour 24, 25, 223, 241, 249
skin cyst 19, 165, 168
skin microbiome 194–5
skin rejuvenation 130, 259–72;
energy-based treatments
266–9; facials 260–1; fillers
264–5; HIFU to achieve an
eyebrow lift 268–9;
hormone replacement
therapy (HRT) 262;
injectable hydrators 265–6;
microneedling 270–2;
'non-surgical' facelifts
267–8; oral isotretinoin
262–3; thread-lifts 269–70;
topical treatments 263
skin structure 13–32; collagen
28; dermis 26–30, 31; hair
follicle 30, 31; hyaluronic
acid (HA) 27–8;
melanocytes 23–5;
sebaceous glands 29–30;
skin colour 24; stem cells
23; stratum corneum 14–21,
18, 26; subcutaneous tissue
31–2, 31; viable epidermis
21–3, 26, 31
skin type, myth of 33–45; dry
skin 38–42; everyone's skin
is fundamentally the same
44; oily skin 34–8; real skin
types 34; sensitive (reactive
skin) 42–4
snipping hair between laser or
IPL treatments 249–51
soaps 17–18, 68, 70–1, 77
sodium lauryl sulphate (SLS)
75–6, 78
solar lentigo (sun freckles) 23,
133
SPF 81, 88–95, 130, 158, 94–5,
263
spinous phase 22

spironolactone 175–7, 181, 199,
247
statins 51, 87, 139
stem cells 23, 153, 274
steroids 79, 107, 115, 135, 138,
150, 167, 179, 215–16, 217,
220, 222, 223; melasma and
224
stratum corneum: acids and 148,
152; acne and 177, 183;
ageing and 50–1;
dermaplaning 253, 254;
dermatitis 217, 219; facial
cleansers/moisturisers and
68, 71, 75–6, 78–9, 80; fats
of 19–20; melasma 222, 224;
rosacea and 203; skincare
ingredients and 112, 113,
114, 115, 116, 117; skincare
products and 97, 98–9; skin
types and 34, 36, 38–9, 41,
42; structure of skin and
13–23, 18, 25, 26, 32;
vitamins and 129, 131, 144
stress 39, 143, 189–90, 192–3,
204, 205, 216
subcutaneous tissue 13, 31, 31,
32
sun exposure 16, 17, 23–5, 31,
34, 37, 39, 47, 48–50, 54, 55,
56, 61, 87–96, 123, 124, 127,
143, 145, 183–4, 198, 199,
202, 203, 204, 207, 210, 216,
223, 225, 227, 231, 233, 263,
272, 275; avoidance 48–9,
101, 124, 211, 222, 272;
hydroquinone and see
hydroquinone; retinoids
and 129–30, 132; sunscreen
and see sunscreen
sunscreen 2, 9, 44, 61, 65, 67, 85,
87–96, 98, 116, 124, 27, 129,
130, 132, 133, 138, 143, 178,
182, 183, 263, 272, 274, 275;
blue light damage 95;

sunscreen – *(Cont.)*
  choosing 89–90; indoors
  96; layer products
  containing SPF 92–3;
  questions 91–3; regulating
  93; removing 89; safety
  93–4; SPF 81, 88–95, 130,
  158, 94–5, 263; using 88–9;
  vitamin D and 90–1
surfactants 17, 68, 220

tazarotene 122, 233
telangiectasia 38, 48,
  145, 204, 205, 210–13,
  223–4
terminal differentiation 22
terminology, skincare 9–10
testosterone 115, 164, 175, 192,
  197, 247
thread-lifts 269–70
threading 132
tissue inhibitors of matrix
  metalloproteinases (TIMPS)
  52–3
toners 1, 7, 35, 97, 100, 131, 158
topical treatments 10, 28, 36, 39,
  61, 79, 93–4, 100, 107–8,
  115, 118, 123, 126, 127,
  134–6, 137, 139, 141–2,
  143–4, 150–1, 154, 156, 179,
  188, 189, 190, 193, 195, 199,
  215, 216, 217, 220; acne and
  168–72; antioxidants 142,
  143–4; retinoids 100,
  128–31, 169, 170, 171, 176,
  181, 188, 233, 244; skin
  rejuvenation and 263;
  tretinoin 123, 127, 129, 178,
  199, 206, 262–3
tranexamic acid (TXA) 222,
  227–8
transepidermal water loss
  (TEWL) 15, 28, 32, 38, 43,
  50, 71, 74, 76, 78, 80, 82,
  148, 156, 177, 183, 203

tretinoin 107, 121–32, 135, 137,
  138, 148, 150, 151, 170,
  171–2, 76, 178, 206, 222,
  223, 224, 233–4, 262–3, 272;
  isotretinoin 176–7, 179–87,
  190, 199, 200, 203, 207, 252,
  262–3
Tri-Luma 135–6
tyrosinase 133, *134*, 138, 225

ultherapy 268–9
UV light 24, 37, 43, 47, 55, 75,
  87–8, 90, 92, 93, 96, 129,
  143, 156, 211, 227, 263
UVB radiation 24, 75, 87, 88, 91,
  92, 93, 129

Varagur, Krithika 111
Vaseline 71, 74, 76, 77, 80, 129,
  155, 156, 179, 208, 216, 220,
  244, 274
viable epidermis 21–6, *26*, 144
vitamin A 100, 121–32, 154, 155,
  171, 182, 184, 262; ageing
  and 124–7; retinoic acid
  122–4; retinoid with other
  skincare products, using
  131–2; topical retinoid
  questions 128–31
vitamin C 28, 102, 108, 116, 132,
  141–5, 153, 221, 241;
  antioxidants and 142–4;
  skincare claims for 145
vitamin D 24, 90–1, 107
vitamin E 37, 142
vitamin K 117
vitiligo 25, 252

water/skin hydration 40
wrinkles 1, 2, 11, 26, 48, 49, 56,
  81, 82, 102, 103, 106, 109,
  124, 125, 126, 145, 151, 208,
  259, 266, 270, 271, 274;
  botulinum toxin and
  234–40, *236*